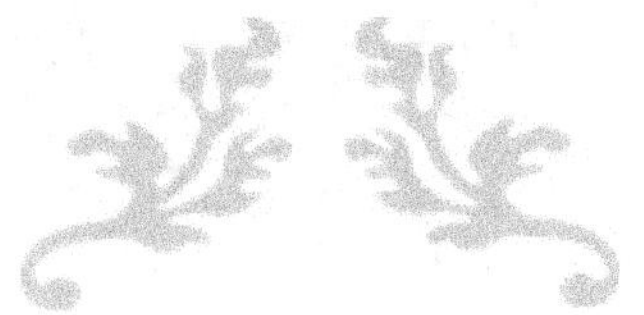

HEALTHY LONGEVITY AND THE BLUE ZONES

Secrets of the World's Longest-Lived Cultures: Living Beyond 100: The Blue Zones Model

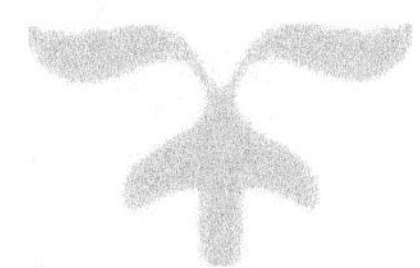

Pedro Agüero Vallejo

Table of Contents

Introduction

Imagine a world where people live to be over 100 years old with health, energy, and a clear purpose. A place where age isn't synonymous with decline, but rather with accumulated wisdom, where a full and active life has no expiration date.

This world is not a figment of fantasy; it exists in so-called "Blue Zones," regions where inhabitants not only outlive the average lifespan, but also maintain an exceptional quality of life.

In "Healthy Longevity and the Blue Zones: Secrets of the World's Longest-Lived Cultures," we will unravel the mysteries behind these communities that have captivated the attention of scientists, doctors, and people from all over the world.

What do places as distant as Ikaria, Greece; Okinawa, Japan; and Nicoya, Costa Rica, have in common? What do their inhabitants do differently to live beyond 100, full of vitality?

This book isn't just an invitation to explore these extraordinary areas; it's a guide to incorporating their principles into our daily lives. Through simple practices, such as natural eating, moderate exercise, social connection, and spirituality, you'll discover how you can transform your approach to health and well-being.

Longevity isn't just a matter of genetics. The latest research reveals that more than 80% of our life expectancy depends on our environment, habits, and lifestyle. This means the power to change is in our hands.

No matter where you live or how old you are, the secrets of the Blue Zones can be the beginning of your own journey to a longer, healthier, and more fulfilling life.

Would you like to know the keys to living beyond 100? In the pages of this book, you'll find inspiration and practical tools to cultivate healthy longevity.

Together, we examine the secrets of the world's longest-living cultures and learn how to apply them so that, like the inhabitants of the Blue Zones, you can enjoy a life full of health and purpose, no matter your age.

The journey to a long life begins here.

Chapter 1:

Secrets of the World's Longest-Living Cultures

The secrets of the world's longest-lived cultures lie in a series of habits and customs that promote health, vitality, and well-being throughout life.

These communities, located in the so-called Blue Zones – Icaria in Greece, Sardinia in Italy, Okinawa in Japan, the Nicoya Peninsula in Costa Rica, and Loma Linda in the United States – have been the subject of numerous studies for their ability to live well into the 100s with an extraordinary quality of life.

Although they are found in different cultural and geographical contexts, they share several factors that appear to be key to their longevity.

One of the most obvious secrets is their diet, which is predominantly plant-based. These cultures consume large amounts of fruits, vegetables, legumes, and whole grains, while meat consumption is limited.

In Okinawa, for example, tofu and purple sweet potatoes are common foods, while in Sardinia, sheep's milk cheese and red wine, rich in antioxidants, are part of the daily diet. This nutrient-dense diet, low in calories and saturated fat, has been linked to a lower incidence of chronic diseases such as diabetes, heart disease, and cancer.

Another pillar of these communities is regular physical activity. Unlike the sedentary lifestyles that predominate in many modern societies, residents of Blue Zones incorporate movement into their daily lives.

In Icaria, people hike through mountainous terrain; in Nicoya, they do physical labor on their land. This isn't intensive exercise, but rather moderate, regular activity that helps maintain a healthy, agile body over the years.

Furthermore, these cultures maintain a strong sense of community and close social relationships. Mutual support among family and friends, as well as a sense of belonging, are fundamental to their emotional well-being.

This sense of community not only reduces stress but also provides a sense of purpose in life, something that is especially relevant in Okinawa, where the concept of ikigai (the reason for living) is deeply rooted in their culture.

Finally, life purpose is a key factor in longevity. Residents of Blue Zones are motivated to continue contributing to their community, which gives them a sense of purpose and satisfaction that significantly prolongs their lives. These secrets, when replicated, offer a valuable lesson on how to live longer and better lives.

Blue Zones are a fascinating phenomenon

The so-called Blue Zones are a fascinating phenomenon that has captured the attention of scientists, doctors, and health enthusiasts around the world. These regions are not merely geographic points on a map; they represent a living laboratory where the secrets of longevity seem to have been unraveled.

The inhabitants of these areas not only reach 100 years of age with surprising frequency, but they do so in exceptional physical and mental health, maintaining a vitality and quality of life that defy expectations.

The five main Blue Zones are distributed throughout the world: Ikaria Island, Greece; Sardinia, Italy; Okinawa, Japan; the Nicoya Peninsula, Costa Rica; and Loma Linda, United States.

Despite the cultural and geographical differences that separate them, they all share one thing in common: their inhabitants live significantly longer than the global average, and many of them surpass the 100-year threshold in perfect health.

This phenomenon has been the subject of extensive demographic and epidemiological studies, as it provides a unique opportunity to understand the key factors behind human longevity.

Why are these regions so special?

What distinguishes Blue Zones isn't a single miraculous factor, but rather a combination of habits and environmental conditions that, together, appear to significantly prolong life. Over the years, researchers have identified several elements shared by these places, which, when replicated, could offer similar benefits to people in other parts of the world. Key factors include:

Plant-based diet: A plant-based diet is one of the most important pillars in the Blue Zones, where longevity is a common characteristic among its inhabitants. In these regions, such as Ikaria in Greece, Okinawa in Japan, and Nicoya in Costa Rica, the diet is primarily focused on plant-based foods, such as legumes, vegetables, fruits, and whole grains.

These foods provide a wealth of essential nutrients and are rich in antioxidants, which play a key role in disease prevention.

One of the highlights of this diet is its low saturated fat content, which comes from the minimal intake of meat and animal products. Instead of relying on red meat or highly processed foods, Blue Zone residents prefer plant-based proteins such as beans, lentils, and tofu.

In Okinawa, for example, purple sweet potatoes are a staple food, while in Sardinia, whole grains and fresh vegetables make up a large part of daily meals. This balanced, fiber-rich diet contributes to metabolic regulation and lower cholesterol levels, two critical factors for cardiovascular health.

A plant-based diet is also rich in antioxidants, which help fight cell damage and reduce inflammation in the body. Antioxidants, found in fruits, vegetables, and whole grains, are associated with a lower incidence of chronic diseases such as cancer, type 2 diabetes, and heart disease. Studies have shown that frequent consumption of these foods protects against premature aging and promotes a better long-term quality of life.

In addition to being a healthy diet, this focus on plant-based foods reflects a deeper connection with the environment. In Blue Zones, local and sustainable agriculture plays a central role, which also contributes to the freshness of the food and a better relationship with nature. The simplicity and naturalness of these meals allow Blue Zone residents to enjoy longer, healthier lives, with fewer diseases and greater overall well-being.

Moderate and consistent physical activity: In Blue Zones, exercise isn't necessarily practiced in gyms or in a structured manner. Instead, people stay active through their daily routines, such as walking, gardening, or doing housework. This type of moderate and regular physical activity has been shown to be extremely beneficial for keeping the body agile and the heart healthy over the years.

A sense of community and social support is a crucial element that distinguishes Blue Zones from the rest of the world, and is closely linked to the longevity and well-being of their inhabitants. In these regions, social connections are deep and meaningful, creating an environment where people live surrounded by family, friends, and neighbors who play an active role in their lives. This strong social fabric not only provides a sense of belonging but also acts as a constant source of emotional and psychological support.

These close, strong relationships are key to reducing stress, one of the biggest factors contributing to a shorter life expectancy in modern societies. Knowing that you have the unconditional support of loved ones in times of need helps mitigate the impact of stress on the body and mind. The feeling of being connected to a community fosters a state of well-being that directly impacts mental health, which, in turn, strengthens physical health.

A notable example is the concept of the "moai" in Okinawa, Japan. The "moai" is a close group of friends formed from childhood and maintained throughout life. These groups provide emotional, financial, and practical support, creating a safety net that helps members face life's challenges.

This model of social support has proven to be a determining factor in the longevity of Okinawans, who have some of the lowest rates of stress-related illnesses.

Overall, the strong sense of community in Blue Zones not only promotes a happier and more balanced life, but also contributes to a longer life expectancy. The sense of belonging to something bigger and having deep and meaningful relationships strengthens emotional and mental health, resulting in a longer, fuller, and more satisfying life.

Life purpose is an essential component in the Blue Zones and plays a significant role in the longevity of its inhabitants. In these regions, people maintain a strong sense of purpose throughout their lives, even into old age, giving them a clear reason to keep going each day. In Okinawa, Japan, this concept is known as "ikigai," which means "the reason for getting up in the morning," while in Nicoya, Costa Rica, it is called "the life plan."

Both terms reflect the importance of having goals, responsibilities, or activities that give a sense of purpose and meaning to their lives.

This sense of purpose not only provides them with daily motivation, but also has a direct impact on their health and well-being. Studies have shown that people who feel they have a clear purpose tend to live longer and healthier lives.

This is partly because purpose in life is linked to lower levels of stress and anxiety, which contribute to better cardiovascular health and greater resistance to disease. Furthermore, a sense of purpose keeps people physically and mentally active, which promotes their overall well-being.

In Blue Zones, residents often continue to play useful roles in their communities or families, which strengthens their social connection and allows them to feel they continue to contribute to something larger than themselves. This focus on transcendence and personal usefulness becomes a driving force that not only lengthens life but also fills it with meaning and satisfaction.

The five places with the highest life expectancy, known as Blue Zones

Icaria, Greece: The secret to a long and healthy life

What is Icaria?

Ikaria is a small island in the Aegean Sea, part of Greece. It is notable for its exceptionally high life expectancy, a very low rate of chronic diseases, and high levels of physical and emotional well-being.

Key factors that make Icaria a Blue Zone:

1. Mediterranean Diet:

Based mainly on vegetables, legumes, fresh fruits, olive oil, whole grains, fish, nuts and wild herbs.

Moderate consumption of local wine, especially red wine, rich in antioxidants.

Low consumption of red meat, processed foods and refined sugars.

2. Natural Physical Activity:

Residents engage in daily physical activity without the need for intense routines. They walk frequently, grow vegetables, fish, and maintain a naturally active lifestyle.

3. **Stress-Free Life:**

The local culture promotes a relaxed lifestyle, avoiding chronic stress.

The daily nap is common, allowing for important physical and mental recovery.

Prioritize personal relationships, adequate rest, and quiet social activities.

4. **Social Connection and Sense of Community:**

Community life is strong, and social interactions are frequent and meaningful.

Strong social support networks contribute to good emotional health and reduce loneliness, an essential factor for longevity.

5. **Purpose of Life (Local Ikigai):**

The people of Icaria find meaning in their daily lives through activities they enjoy, such as farming, cooking for their families, and spending time with friends.

The sense of purpose is maintained throughout life, even into advanced age.

Health outcomes:

Very low incidence of cardiovascular disease, diabetes and cancer.

High proportion of people over 90 years of age with a good quality of life.

Low rates of dementia and cognitive impairments, attributed to a diet rich in antioxidants, regular physical activity, and ongoing cognitive stimulation through social interactions.

Icaria exemplifies how factors such as a healthy diet, an active lifestyle, low exposure to stress, and strong community ties directly contribute to healthy longevity.

Sardinia, Italy: The place where men live as long as women

What makes Sardinia special?

Sardinia, especially its mountainous Barbagia region, is known worldwide for its astonishing number of healthy centenarians. Unlike other parts of the world, men here have a similar life expectancy to women, which is exceptional worldwide.

Key features that make Sardinia a Blue Zone:

1. Sardinian diet, rich in antioxidants

A diet based on local produce such as fresh fruits and vegetables, whole grains, legumes (especially fava beans), sheep cheese (pecorino), goat's milk, nuts, extra virgin olive oil, and local wine rich in antioxidants (especially Cannonau wine, with its high levels of polyphenols).

Moderate consumption of meat, mainly from free-range animals.

This locally adapted Mediterranean diet reduces inflammation, fights heart disease, and contributes to excellent overall health.

2. Daily and constant physical activity

The inhabitants, especially the Sardinian shepherds, lead a naturally active life, constantly hiking through mountainous terrain as they herd sheep and goats daily.

This continuous physical activity improves the cardiovascular system, strengthens bones and joints, maintains a healthy weight, and prevents diseases associated with a sedentary lifestyle.

3. Strong sense of community and family connection

Sardinian communities are particularly close-knit; family and neighborly relationships play a crucial role in emotional well-being.

Intergenerational family life ensures constant social support, helping to maintain good mental health and reducing the incidence of depression and anxiety in later life.

4. Equality in longevity between men and women

Unlike other regions of the world, in Sardinia men have a similar life expectancy to women.

This is primarily a result of an active lifestyle and healthy diet, which particularly protect men against cardiovascular disease, one of the leading causes of male mortality globally.

5. Purpose and sense of identity

The Sardinians maintain a strong sense of cultural identity, rooted in their traditions and activities that give them meaning (herding, agriculture, artisanal food production and local products).

This deep sense of purpose (known locally as a "life plan") helps maintain daily motivation and vitality well into old age.

Observed health benefits:

High proportion of people who reach and exceed 100 years of age, maintaining autonomy and quality of life.

Very low prevalence of heart disease, diabetes and cognitive impairment.

Better overall levels of physical and emotional well-being compared to other regions.

Sardinia. It is a clear example of how the combination of a balanced diet, daily physical activity, strong social connection, and a clear life purpose can produce extraordinary longevity.

Okinawa, Japan: The Eastern Secret of Longevity

Okinawa is a Japanese archipelago known worldwide for having one of the highest rates of centenarians, with a high quality of life and excellent physical and mental health.

Key features that make Okinawa a Blue Zone:

1. Traditional Okinawan Diet:

Based on fresh, natural foods such as purple sweet potatoes, rich in antioxidants and fiber, which constitute the main caloric base of your diet.

Regular consumption of tofu and other soy products, important sources of vegetable protein that promote bone and hormonal health.

Frequent consumption of fresh fish and seaweed, rich in Omega-3, vital for maintaining cardiovascular health.

The diet is low in saturated fat, refined sugar, and red meat.

2. Principle of the "Hara Hachi Bu" rule:

It is a conscious practice of eating until you feel 80% satisfied, which avoids caloric excesses and prevents metabolic diseases, promoting a healthy weight in the long term.

3. Ikigai: Having a purpose in life:

The concept of Ikigai ("the reason one gets up each morning") is fundamental in Okinawa.

Residents cultivate a strong sense of purpose, whether it's gardening, teaching martial arts, community activities, or caring for their families.

This generates a deep motivation that improves your emotional and mental health.

4. Moai: Strong community ties:

Moai is a cultural tradition that involves forming groups of friends to provide social, emotional, and economic support throughout life.

These strong social networks protect against depression, anxiety, and social isolation, promoting an emotionally healthy and resilient life.

5. Physically active and daily life:

Okinawans stay naturally active, engaging in gardening, tai chi, traditional dancing, walking, and other gentle but consistent forms of physical exercise.

This promotes strong bones, toned muscles, and good cardiovascular and cognitive health well into old age.

Observed health outcomes:

A high proportion of people who live to be over 100 years old are mentally alert and physically independent.

Low rates of heart disease, cancer, osteoporosis, diabetes, and degenerative diseases such as Alzheimer's.

Excellent emotional well-being due to the combination of purpose, balanced nutrition, and strong community life.

OkinawaIt is an excellent example of how a balanced diet, an active lifestyle, having a clear reason for living (ikigai), and strong community ties (moai) can help people live longer, but above all, with a higher quality of life.

Nicoya, Costa Rica: Longevity in the heart of Central America

The Nicoya Peninsula is globally recognized for the impressive longevity of its inhabitants, who enjoy active, happy, and healthy lives, easily reaching old age with vigor and clarity.

Key factors that make Nicoya a Blue Zone:

1. Simple and Nutritious Diet:

The basic diet in Nicoya is simple, based on local foods such as corn, beans, and fresh tropical fruits (papaya, mango, banana).

Corn and beans combined provide a complete source of plant-based protein, complex carbohydrates, and fiber, which help maintain cardiovascular and digestive health.

Reduce consumption of red meat, processed foods, and refined sugars, promoting a diet rich in antioxidants and essential nutrients.

2. Consumption of Mineral-Rich Water:

The water in Nicoya is rich in calcium and magnesium, essential minerals that contribute to strong bones, reduce osteoporosis, and improve cardiovascular health.

3. Daily Physical Activity:

Residents regularly engage in natural physical activities such as walking long distances daily, working in the fields, farming, livestock, gardening, and housework.

This regular physical exercise strengthens muscles and bones and significantly improves cardiovascular health.

4. Strong Family and Social Connection:

Family and close friends play an essential role in the daily lives of Nicoya residents.

The social system offers constant emotional support, significantly reducing stress, anxiety, and depression.

Older adults remain integrated into communities and homes, playing active roles in educating and guiding younger generations.

5. Plan of Life and Spiritual Faith:

The inhabitants of Nicoya maintain a clear purpose in their lives ("life plan"), which includes family commitment, active participation in communities, and daily work that provides personal satisfaction.

In addition, they maintain a strong spiritual or religious faith, which provides them with comfort, resilience, and hope in difficult times.

Observed health outcomes:

High proportion of people over 90 and centenarians who live independent and active lives.

Low levels of cardiovascular disease, type 2 diabetes, and dementia.

Better mental health thanks to consistent social support and a purpose-driven life.

Nicoya. It teaches us how a simple life, based on local foods, daily physical labor, strong family and social ties, along with a clear purpose and deep spirituality, can translate into extraordinary longevity and quality of life.

Loma Linda: A special community in the middle of North America

Loma Linda, California, is a notable exception in the United States: it is home to a community of Seventh-day Adventists who enjoy a significantly longer lifespan than the North American average, maintaining an excellent quality of life even into old age.

Key factors that make Loma Linda a Blue Zone:

1. Vegetarian or Plant-Based Diet:

Most Adventist residents of Loma Linda follow a predominantly vegetarian or vegan diet.

They consume fruits, vegetables, whole grains, legumes, nuts and seeds, foods naturally rich in fiber, antioxidants and essential micronutrients.

This diet prevents heart disease, type 2 diabetes, cancer, and obesity, contributing to a better quality of life and life expectancy.

2. Regular Practice of Weekly Rest (Sabbath):

Every week, Adventists celebrate the Sabbath (Saturday) as a day dedicated exclusively to physical, mental, and spiritual rest.

This habit helps reduce the stress accumulated during the week, improves emotional health, and allows for deep recovery, promoting a healthy balance between work and rest.

3. Active Social and Community Life:

In Loma Linda, the community regularly participates in religious, educational, and recreational activities, maintaining strong ties and solid support networks.

This community integration protects against social isolation, promoting good mental and emotional health.

4. Constant and Moderate Physical Exercise:

Residents regularly engage in moderate physical activity, such as daily walking, swimming, cycling, and other outdoor recreational activities.

In addition, many older Adventists continue to be actively involved in volunteer and community activities, which keeps them physically and mentally active.

5. Vital Purpose and Spirituality:

Faith and spirituality play a central role in the lives of Adventists, providing a clear existential purpose that fosters optimism and resilience in the face of difficulties.

This spiritual approach is linked to a positive attitude, emotional stability, and a general sense of satisfaction with life.

Observed health outcomes:

Loma Linda residents live an average of 7 to 10 years longer than the average U.S. population.

Low incidence of chronic diseases such as diabetes, hypertension, cardiovascular disease and certain types of cancer.

High quality of life and emotional well-being in later life due to a strong sense of purpose and community connection.

Loma Linda. It is an excellent example of how a balanced lifestyle that includes a healthy diet, regular rest, moderate physical exercise, and a strong spiritual and social connection can result in greater longevity and overall well-being.

Summary on blue zones

Icaria, Greece. Known as the place where people "forget to die," Ikaria is a small Aegean island that has become synonymous with longevity. Its inhabitants have one of the highest rates of centenarians in the world, with a very low incidence of chronic diseases such as cancer and heart disease. What makes Ikaria exceptional is not only the longevity of its population, but also the quality of life they maintain into old age, maintaining high levels of mental and physical activity.

One of the key secrets of the Icarians is their Mediterranean diet, rich in olive oil, legumes, fresh vegetables, and fruits, which provides an abundant source of antioxidants and healthy fats. This balanced diet, combined with moderate red wine consumption, helps protect the heart and reduce the risk of inflammatory and chronic diseases.

However, diet isn't the only determining factor. Icarians lead a relaxed lifestyle that prioritizes rest and sleep, with a culture that favors daily siestas and a relaxed approach to everyday tasks.

This stress-free lifestyle, combined with light, consistent physical activity, such as walking or gardening, contributes to their overall well-being and longevity. In Icaria, the balance between body and mind, reinforced by strong community and family ties, is an effective formula for living longer and better.

Sardinia, Italy. In the mountainous region of Sardinia, a globally unusual phenomenon occurs: men achieve a life expectancy similar to that of women, something uncommon in other parts of the world. This shared longevity between genders has been the subject of studies due to the lifestyle habits characteristic of Sardinian shepherds, who walk long distances daily across rugged terrain. This constant, moderate but regular physical activity is one of the key factors contributing to their cardiovascular health and longevity.

The diet of Sardinians also plays a fundamental role in their longevity. It is based primarily on local products, such as sheep's milk cheese, rich in healthy fats and essential nutrients, and red wine, which contains high levels of antioxidants, particularly polyphenols.

These compounds help combat cellular aging and protect against chronic diseases, such as cardiovascular disease and cancer.

In addition to its diet and physical activity, family and community ties are strong in this region, providing an emotionally supportive environment that also contributes to its overall well-being. The combination of a nutrient-dense diet, consistent physical activity, and a close-knit social environment makes Sardinia one of the most studied and admired Blue Zones in the world.

Okinawa, Japan Okinawa is internationally recognized as home to some of the world's longest-lived people. Residents of this Japanese island enjoy an exceptional life expectancy, which has sparked the interest of scientists and health experts.

One of the keys to this longevity is their diet, which includes nutrient-dense, low-calorie foods like tofu, fish, and purple sweet potatoes, known for their high antioxidant and fiber content. This diet contributes to the low incidence of chronic diseases like diabetes and heart disease among the Okinawan population.

However, Okinawan longevity is not solely due to diet. A crucial factor is their close social support network and the strong sense of community they maintain throughout their lives. Okinawans develop deep and lasting interpersonal relationships, which provide them with a solid emotional foundation. The concept of "moai," a network of friends who support each other throughout life, is an example of how social support can influence well-being.

Furthermore, Okinawans possess a clearly defined sense of purpose, known as "ikigai," or "the reason to get up in the morning." This sense of having a clear purpose in life, which persists even into old age, provides them with daily motivation and a reason to stay active. Both "ikigai" and "moai" are fundamental to their emotional health, reducing stress levels and promoting a longer, more fulfilling life.

The combination of these factors makes Okinawa a model of sustainable longevity, where diet, life purpose, and social relationships form the foundation of a healthy and long life.

Nicoya, Costa Rica. On the Nicoya Peninsula, residents enjoy a long life thanks to a simple lifestyle and a close connection with nature. The people of this region lead active, healthy lives, fostered by a traditional diet based on corn, beans, and fresh fruits, foods that provide them with balanced nutrition rich in fiber, plant proteins, and antioxidants. This diet, low in processed meats and high in essential nutrients, contributes to a reduction in chronic diseases and a longer life.

Another crucial factor for longevity in Nicoya is the quality of the local water, which is rich in calcium and magnesium, two minerals essential for bone health. Thanks to this, the region's residents have a lower incidence of bone fractures and diseases related to bone density, allowing them to maintain active mobility even into advanced age.

Family connection is another essential aspect of life in Nicoya. Family relationships are very close, and elders occupy a respected place within their communities, which strengthens their emotional well-being and provides them with a sense of belonging and support.

Furthermore, daily physical labor remains part of the routine of many Nicoyans, which, along with their diet and natural environment, helps keep them active and physically fit throughout their lives. This lifestyle, which integrates nature, nutrition, and personal relationships, makes Nicoya one of the longest-lived and healthiest Blue Zones in the world.

Loma Linda, United States. This Adventist community in California is distinguished by its focus on holistic health and spirituality, which has contributed to its reputation as a Blue Zone. Seventh-day Adventists living in Loma Linda embrace a lifestyle that prioritizes disease prevention and physical and mental well-being.

One of the pillars of their longevity is their vegetarian diet, rich in fruits, vegetables, legumes, and nuts, which provides them with balanced nutrition and is low in saturated fat. By avoiding meat, processed foods, alcohol, and tobacco, Adventists significantly reduce their risk of chronic diseases such as cancer and heart disease.

In addition to their focus on diet, Adventists practice weekly rest through the Sabbath, a day dedicated to spiritual reflection, rest, and family activities. This day of rest not only helps reduce accumulated stress but also fosters greater connection with community and their faith. The combination of a healthy lifestyle and a strong focus on spirituality and community contributes to a more balanced life, reducing the impact of stressors and promoting overall well-being.

The commitment to physical and spiritual health at Loma Linda has allowed many of its residents to enjoy long and full lives, demonstrating how a life focused on prevention, moderation, and connection with deep values can have a direct impact on longevity.

The science behind Blue Zones

The science behind Blue Zones. Has revealed that longevity is not simply a matter of genetics, but is profoundly influenced by a combination of lifestyle habits, behavioral patterns, and environmental factors. Over years of research in regions such as Ikaria in Greece, Okinawa in Japan, and Nicoya in Costa Rica, scientists have identified a series of common characteristics that appear to be key to helping residents of these areas live longer and with a better quality of life.

One of the most notable findings is that people in Blue Zones follow a plant-based diet, rich in fruits, vegetables, legumes, and whole grains, and low in processed foods and red meat.

This diet not only reduces the incidence of chronic diseases, such as cardiovascular disease and cancer, but also promotes better mental and physical health.

Foods consumed in these regions are full of antioxidants, healthy fats, and fiber, which contribute to the prevention of aging-related diseases.

In addition to diet, another key factor is the moderate but consistent level of physical activity that Blue Zone residents engage in daily. Unlike modern societies, where exercise is often structured, in Blue Zones, physical activity is naturally integrated into daily life, such as walking, gardening, or caring for animals. This active lifestyle helps maintain good cardiovascular and muscular health, allowing people to remain independent and agile even into advanced age.

The sense of community and interpersonal relationships also play a crucial role in longevity. Studies show that emotional support from family and friends is a powerful source of well-being.

In Okinawa, for example, social groups known as "moai" form in childhood and provide a support network throughout life. These deep social ties not only reduce stress but also strengthen emotional health, which directly impacts longevity.

Finally, people in the Blue Zones have a clear life purpose, an essential element that gives them daily motivation to stay active and mentally engaged. Whether through the concept of "ikigai" in Japan or the "life plan" in Nicoya, this sense of purpose provides meaning to their lives, helping them face challenges with a positive and resilient outlook.

Although not all of the Blue Zones' elements can be replicated elsewhere, many of their principles are universal and can be adopted to improve the quality of life anywhere in the world. Healthy eating, moderate exercise, strong social relationships, and a sense of purpose are lessons anyone can incorporate into their lives to live longer and better.

Ultimately, Blue Zones are not just enclaves of longevity, but an inspiring model for caring for our body, mind, and spirit, and thus enjoying a long, healthy, and meaningful life.

Social factors that promote longevity.

The social factors that promote longevity are deeply intertwined with the interpersonal relationships and sense of community that people develop throughout their lives. In Blue Zones, one of the key elements is the strong social support network that surrounds residents, providing them with a sense of belonging and emotional connection.

Multigenerational families living together, close friends, and neighbors who look out for each other are common features in these regions. This social network not only provides physical support in times of need, but also emotional support that reduces stress, one of the main factors contributing to premature aging and chronic diseases.

Another important social factor is the inclusion of older adults in the daily life of their communities. Unlike many modern societies, where older adults are often marginalized, in Blue Zones, older adults play active and valuable roles within their families and communities.

They are respected for their wisdom and experience, which gives them a strong sense of purpose, a key factor in maintaining a mentally active and emotionally balanced life.

Furthermore, community celebrations and rituals are an integral part of social life in these regions, where people gather regularly to share food, stories, and moments of reflection. These frequent interactions strengthen social ties and create a cohesive community that fosters happiness and overall well-being. The combination of these social factors not only improves quality of life but has also been shown to prolong life expectancy, demonstrating the importance of human relationships in overall well-being.

Food and diet in the blue zones.

The diet and nutrition of Blue Zones play a fundamental role in the longevity of their inhabitants. These regions share a dietary approach based primarily on plant-based products, which translates into diets rich in fruits, vegetables, legumes, and whole grains, while the consumption of meat and processed foods is limited.

This type of diet, characterized by its abundance of antioxidants, fiber, and healthy fats, is directly linked to a reduction in chronic diseases such as diabetes, cancer, and heart disease.

In Icaria, Greece, for example, the Mediterranean diet based on olive oil, legumes, and fresh vegetables is an essential component of longevity, while in Okinawa, Japan, foods like tofu, fish, and purple sweet potatoes are the pillars of a diet that promotes cellular health and combats aging. Similarly, in Nicoya, Costa Rica, local corn, beans, and fruits provide a simple yet balanced diet rich in plant-based proteins and essential nutrients.

Another key aspect of the Blue Zone diet is moderation. Small portions and avoiding overeating are common, helping to maintain a healthy weight and prevent metabolic diseases. Furthermore, the focus on fresh, local foods, along with minimal consumption of processed products, reduces exposure to harmful substances such as preservatives and added sugars, promoting optimal long-term health.

Together, a plant-based diet and food moderation are key elements for longevity in the Blue Zones. These eating habits not only contribute to physical health but also encourage a more conscious and balanced lifestyle, focused on disease prevention and promoting a long, healthy life.

The impact of community and social relationships.

The impact of community and social relationships is one of the most influential factors in the longevity and well-being of individuals, especially in Blue Zones. People living in these regions enjoy long lives not only due to their eating and exercise habits, but also due to the quality and depth of their social connections.

Being surrounded by a strong network of family, friends, and neighbors who provide emotional and physical support significantly contributes to stress reduction, improves mental health, and strengthens resilience in the face of life's challenges.

In many modern societies, isolation and loneliness have become public health problems, linked to a higher incidence of chronic diseases and reduced life expectancy. However, in Blue Zones, residents value the importance of interpersonal relationships as an essential aspect of their daily lives.

In Okinawa, Japan, for example, the concept of "moai" – small groups of friends who support each other throughout life – strengthens a sense of belonging and emotional security, reducing the risk of depression and other mental health problems.

Intergenerational family relationships are also common in these regions, where older adults continue to be an active part of the family and community. This respect and appreciation for the elderly not only provides them with a strong sense of purpose but also creates an environment in which they feel supported and useful, contributing to a longer, healthier life.

The constant social support experienced in Blue Zones allows individuals to cope with life's stress and difficulties more easily, knowing they have the support of those around them. This support network fosters a sense of security, happiness, and well-being that has been shown to directly impact longevity.

So, social relationships and a sense of community not only promote a more fulfilling life, but are also essential components for living longer and with a better quality of life.

Chapter 2.
Discover the Keys to a Healthy and Longer Life

Discovering the keys to a healthy and long life means understanding that longevity is not just a matter of genetics, but depends largely on the lifestyle habits adopted over time.

Studies conducted in Blue Zones, where residents enjoy exceptionally long and healthy lives, reveal a number of key factors that anyone can implement to improve their quality of life and increase their life expectancy.

One of the key elements is a balanced, predominantly plant-based diet. People in Blue Zones consume diets rich in fruits, vegetables, legumes, and whole grains, with little meat and almost no processed foods.

This diet is not only rich in antioxidants and essential nutrients, but also contributes to the prevention of chronic diseases such as diabetes, cancer, and heart disease. Portion moderation and respect for the natural cycles of hunger and satiety also play an important role in metabolic health.

Another essential key is regular physical activity. Unlike modern approaches to exercise, in the Blue Zones, physical activity is naturally integrated into everyday life.

People walk, grow their own food, and perform household chores that keep them moving throughout the day.

This type of moderate but consistent exercise not only strengthens the body but also improves cardiovascular health and keeps energy levels high even into old age.

Social support and a sense of community are also crucial. In these regions, people maintain strong ties with their families, friends, and neighbors, providing them with a solid network of emotional support.

Studies have shown that close interpersonal relationships reduce stress levels, improve mental health, and contribute to overall well-being that promotes longevity. Feeling part of a community and knowing that others support you is a factor that positively impacts emotional and physical health.

Furthermore, a sense of purpose is a powerful key to a long life. In Blue Zones, older adults are not marginalized but instead play active roles in their communities and families.

This sense of purpose—whether through "ikigai" in Okinawa or the "life plan" in Nicoya—gives them a reason to stay active and mentally engaged, reducing the risk of neurodegenerative diseases and fostering a positive attitude toward aging.

Finally, stress reduction is essential for a long life. People in Blue Zones practice simple and effective ways to manage stress, such as taking daily naps, engaging in relaxing activities, or participating in spiritual rituals.

Adequate rest, both physical and mental, is essential to keeping the body and mind in balance, allowing you to face life's challenges with greater resilience.

Together, these factors—healthy eating, physical activity, social support, purpose in life, and stress management—are the keys to a long and well-being life. These principles are applicable anywhere, and by adopting them, it's possible not only to live longer, but also to enjoy a more fulfilling and satisfying life.

The importance of moderate and constant exercise.

The importance of moderate and constant exercise. Its value lies in its ability to improve physical, mental, and emotional health throughout life. Unlike modern approaches, which often emphasize intense workouts in short bursts, in Blue Zones, where people live longer and better lives, exercise is incorporated naturally into their daily routines. This type of moderate but consistent physical activity has numerous proven benefits that promote a long and healthy life.

Moderate exercise includes simple activities such as walking, biking, gardening, or doing housework, all of which keep the body moving without requiring extreme exertion. This approach is not only more accessible to people of all ages, but also reduces the risk of injury and exhaustion that can be more common with high-intensity workouts.

Furthermore, by becoming part of your daily routine, moderate exercise becomes a sustainable, long-term habit, which is essential for maintaining an active lifestyle.

One of the most important benefits of moderate, consistent exercise is its impact on cardiovascular health. Activities such as walking or stair climbing stimulate blood circulation and strengthen the heart, reducing the risk of heart disease, one of the leading causes of death worldwide. By keeping the heart active, exercise helps control

cholesterol and blood pressure levels, improving the overall health of the cardiovascular system.

Furthermore, regular exercise has a significant impact on
metabolic health. Regular movement helps regulate blood
sugar levels, which is essential for preventing or managing
diseases like type 2 diabetes. Moderate physical activity
also contributes to maintaining a healthy weight, which
reduces the risk of developing metabolic problems and
helps maintain the body's energy balance.

Regarding mental health, regular exercise acts as a powerful mood regulator. Studies have shown that physical activity releases endorphins, hormones associated with feelings of well-being and happiness. This release of endorphins helps reduce stress and anxiety levels and is also a
key factor in preventing depression.

Regular exercise also improves cognitive function and
contributes to greater mental clarity, which can protect
against neurodegenerative diseases such as Alzheimer's.

Another important aspect of moderate, consistent exercise
is its impact on muscle and bone strength. Staying active
regularly improves bone density and muscle strength,
which is crucial for preventing fractures and falls, especially in old age. People who engage in gentle but consistent exercise such as walking or yoga experience less
muscle loss over time, allowing them to remain mobile
and active even in old age.

Finally, moderate exercise also promotes better sleep
quality. People who are physically active during the day

tend to sleep better at night, which improves the body's rest and recovery. Restful sleep is essential for overall health, as it allows the body to regenerate and the brain to process the day's information.

Moderate, consistent exercise is a powerful tool for maintaining good health throughout life. It not only improves cardiovascular and metabolic function, but also strengthens muscles and bones, protects mental health, and improves sleep quality.

The key to its success lies in its sustainability: as a natural part of daily life, this type of exercise doesn't require great effort but offers great long-term rewards, contributing to a longer, healthier, and more fulfilling life.

The plant-based diet and its influence on health.

The importance of moderate and constant exercise. Its value lies in its ability to improve physical, mental, and emotional health throughout life. Unlike modern approaches, which often emphasize intense workouts in short bursts, in Blue Zones, where people live longer and better lives, exercise is incorporated naturally into their daily routines. This type of moderate but consistent physical activity has numerous proven benefits that promote a long and healthy life.

Moderate exercise includes simple activities such as walking, biking, gardening, or doing housework, all of which keep the body moving without requiring extreme exertion. This approach is not only more accessible to people of all ages, but it also reduces the risk of injury and burnout, which can be more common with high-intensity workouts. Furthermore, by becoming part of a daily routine, moderate exercise becomes a sustainable long-term habit, which is essential for maintaining an active lifestyle.

One of the most important benefits of moderate, consistent exercise is its impact on cardiovascular health. Activities such as walking or stair climbing stimulate blood circulation and strengthen the heart, reducing the risk of heart disease, one of the leading causes of death worldwide.

By keeping the heart active, exercise helps control cholesterol and blood pressure levels, improving the overall health of the cardiovascular system.

Furthermore, regular exercise has a significant impact on metabolic health. Regular movement helps regulate blood sugar levels, which is essential for preventing or managing diseases like type 2 diabetes.

Moderate physical activity also contributes to maintaining a healthy weight, which reduces the risk of developing metabolic problems and helps maintain the body's energy balance.

Regarding mental health, consistent exercise acts as a powerful mood regulator. Studies have shown that physical activity releases endorphins, hormones associated with feelings of well-being and happiness. This release of endorphins helps reduce stress and anxiety levels and is also a key factor in preventing depression. Consistent exercise also improves cognitive function and contributes to greater mental clarity, which can protect against neurodegenerative diseases such as Alzheimer's.

Another important aspect of moderate, consistent exercise is its impact on muscle and bone strength. Staying active regularly improves bone density and muscle strength, which is crucial for preventing fractures and falls, especially in old age.

People who engage in gentle but consistent exercise such as walking or yoga experience less muscle loss over time, allowing them to remain mobile and active even in old age.

Moderate exercise also promotes better sleep quality, and its impact on the ability to achieve deep rest is widely recognized by scientific studies. People who stay physically active during the day, whether through walking, gardening, or everyday activities that involve movement, tend to experience more restful sleep at night.

This improvement in sleep quality is due to several factors involving both the body and the mind, as physical activity regulates sleep cycles, reduces stress, and helps the body relax more easily at the end of the day.

One of the reasons exercise promotes better sleep is because it helps reduce stress and anxiety levels. Chronic stress is one of the main factors contributing to sleep problems such as insomnia.

Moderate physical activity acts as a way to release accumulated tension, allowing the body and mind to relax at the end of the day.

Additionally, exercise promotes the production of endorphins, hormones that improve mood and reduce feelings of anxiety. This calming effect not only improves the ability to fall asleep but also allows for deeper, uninterrupted rest.

Restful sleep is essential for overall health, as it's when the body carries out vital regeneration and recovery processes. During deep sleep, the body works to repair damaged muscle tissue, strengthen the immune system, and regulate hormones that control hunger and metabolism.

Lack of adequate sleep can interfere with these processes, increasing the risk of chronic diseases such as obesity, diabetes, and heart disease. People who engage in moderate exercise tend to spend more time in the deeper stages of sleep, which improves these recovery processes.

Additionally, physical exercise helps regulate circadian rhythms, the body's internal cycles that control sleep and wakefulness.

Exposure to natural light and movement during the day helps the body establish a healthy circadian rhythm, making it easier to fall asleep at night. People who lead active lifestyles often experience less difficulty falling asleep and fewer awakenings during the night, resulting in greater sleep efficiency.

The benefits of exercise on sleep also have cumulative effects.

The more regular physical activity is, the more sleep patterns stabilize, which can lead to continued improvements in sleep quality. This is especially important for older adults, who may experience more sleep problems due to natural changes in circadian rhythms and reduced daily physical activity.

By maintaining a constant level of movement, even moderate, it is possible to counteract some of these effects and enjoy more restful sleep.

Thus, moderate and consistent exercise is a powerful tool for maintaining good health throughout life. Not only does it improve cardiovascular and metabolic function, but it also strengthens muscles and bones, protects mental health, and improves sleep quality. The key to its success lies in its sustainability: as a natural part of daily life, this type of exercise doesn't require great effort but offers great long-term rewards, contributing to a longer, healthier, and more fulfilling life.

The connection between spirituality and longevity.

The connection between spirituality and longevity is a topic that has sparked growing interest in the fields of science and health. Numerous studies have shown that people who practice some form of spirituality or have a strong belief in something beyond the material tend to live longer and with a better quality of life.

Although the exact mechanisms of this connection are not fully understood, there are several key factors that explain how spirituality can influence longevity, both physically and emotionally.

First, spirituality offers a sense of purpose and meaning in life, which has been directly linked to increased longevity. In Blue Zones, such as Okinawa, Japan, the concept of "ikigai" (the reason for getting up in the morning) is central to the emotional well-being and longevity of its residents.

Having a clear purpose, whether religious, spiritual, or based on a personal mission, helps people maintain a positive focus, even during difficult times, and gives them a reason to stay active and mentally engaged over the years.

This sense of purpose and direction has been shown to reduce stress, one of the main factors contributing to chronic disease and premature aging.

Spiritual practice is also often linked to daily routines that promote peace of mind and well-being. Activities such as prayer, meditation, yoga, and personal reflection help reduce stress and anxiety levels.

These practices promote inner calm and help manage emotions in a more balanced way, which has a direct impact on physical health. Chronic stress has been linked to a range of health problems, including heart disease, hypertension, and immune disorders.

By reducing stress, spirituality acts as a buffer against these risk factors, promoting a longer, healthier life.

Furthermore, spiritual or religious people often participate in faith communities, which provide them with a strong social support network. A sense of belonging and close interpersonal relationships are essential components for a long and healthy life. Faith communities often offer emotional support, social connection, and opportunities for service, which strengthens the bonds between individuals and provides a solid support system.

Close and meaningful relationships, as observed in the Blue Zones, not only reduce isolation and loneliness, but also promote longevity by providing a network that supports people through difficult times.

Another crucial aspect is that many spiritual practices promote a balanced and moderate life. For example, Seventh-day Adventists in the Loma Linda Blue Zone in the United States follow a predominantly vegetarian diet and avoid alcohol and tobacco.

These spiritual practices, which advocate moderation and self-care, not only protect physical health but also promote longevity. People who follow these rules tend to have a lower risk of chronic diseases and enjoy a better quality of life.

Spirituality fosters a resilient attitude toward life's challenges, providing people with a broader and more serene perspective on suffering and difficulties. Those who practice some form of spirituality, whether through religion or a personal search for meaning, tend to view problems and difficult times as opportunities for growth and learning rather than insurmountable obstacles.

This ability to face adversity with calm and strength is due to several key reasons that are deeply connected to the nature of spirituality.

First, spirituality offers a framework that helps people contextualize suffering within a larger narrative. In many spiritual and religious traditions, suffering is not seen as a punishment or a meaningless negative event, but as an integral part of life that serves a purpose.

This belief allows individuals to face difficulties with greater acceptance, knowing that these experiences, although painful, can lead to greater understanding, empathy, and personal growth.

For example, in Christianity, suffering is often associated with redemption or spiritual development, while in Buddhism it is seen as an opportunity to practice compassion and non-attachment.

Furthermore, spirituality provides a sense of connection to something greater than oneself, whether a deity, the universe, or a transcendental spiritual force. This belief that there is a higher purpose behind life and its challenges provides a sense of comfort and emotional stability.

Spiritual people tend to feel that they are not alone in their struggle and that, in some way, what they face has meaning that may not be immediately apparent, but is part of a larger plan. This belief fosters a resilient attitude because it reduces the sense of hopelessness and loss of control that often accompanies personal crises.

The Spiritual practice also often includes effective methods for managing stress, such as meditation, prayer, or reflection. These activities promote inner calm and allow people to process their emotions in a more balanced way.

The ability to connect with oneself or a higher power through these practices creates a sense of peace and acceptance that is crucial for dealing with difficult situations.

Furthermore, these moments of introspection allow people to observe their problems from a more serene and objective perspective, which helps them avoid impulsive or destructive reactions to suffering.

Another important aspect is that spirituality often encourages the practice of gratitude and focusing on the positive, even in the midst of adversity. Many spiritual people develop the ability to find meaning in the small things in life, which helps them maintain a positive attitude even in times of difficulty.

This focus on gratitude allows individuals to recognize that, despite challenges, there is always something valuable to be grateful for, which helps them cope better during times of crisis.

Spiritual resilience is also deeply connected to faith in an existence beyond physical life or in a transcendental purpose that gives meaning to life. This belief reduces the fear of suffering and, in particular, the fear of death, which is one of the greatest sources of human anxiety.

By understanding death as part of a cycle or as a transition to something else, spiritual people experience less anxiety about their own mortality, allowing them to live more serenely and accept challenges as a natural part of existence.

Finally, spiritual community plays a fundamental role in developing resilience. People who participate in faith communities often have a strong network of emotional and practical support to turn to during difficult times.

This network provides comfort, understanding, and help when it's most needed, making it easier to overcome challenges. The sense of belonging to a community that shares the same beliefs and values also strengthens personal resilience, as people don't feel isolated in their suffering.

Whether through belief in an afterlife or in the existence of a higher purpose, this perspective reduces anxiety and fear of death, which can lead to greater inner peace and emotional stability. People who manage stress and adversity more effectively tend to have fewer health problems and, therefore, live longer.

In short, the connection between spirituality and longevity is multifaceted. Spirituality provides a sense of purpose, promotes stress reduction, fosters close social relationships, and advocates for a moderate lifestyle—all factors linked to a longer lifespan.

By integrating spiritual practices into everyday life, whether through religious faith or a personal sense of connection to something greater, it is possible to improve emotional, mental, and physical health, which can result in a longer, more fulfilling, and balanced life.

Adequate rest as an essential part of well-being.

Adequate rest is an essential part of physical, mental, and emotional well-being and plays a pivotal role in maintaining a healthy life. Often underestimated in modern societies, where fast-paced life and daily responsibilities take center stage, rest is a time when the body and mind regenerate, allowing both to function optimally.

Lack of adequate rest not only affects daily energy and mood, but is also linked to a number of serious health problems, including heart disease, metabolic disorders, and a weakened immune system.

One of the most important aspects of rest is restorative sleep. During sleep, the body enters a state of profound regeneration. In the deepest stages of sleep, known as slow-wave sleep and REM (rapid eye movement) sleep, the body repairs tissues, strengthens muscles, consolidates memory, and balances hormones that regulate hunger, stress, and metabolism.

Inadequate or interrupted sleep can interfere with these processes, leading to a decrease in concentration, decision-making, and emotional management. In the long term, a lack of adequate sleep is associated with an increased risk of developing chronic diseases, such as type 2 diabetes, hypertension, and cardiovascular problems.

Mental rest is equally crucial for well-being. In today's world, many people experience cognitive overload due to excessive stimulation, whether through work, social media, or technology. This can cause mental fatigue, a condition in which the brain struggles to process information and maintain focus.

Resting gives the mind a chance to disconnect from daily demands, allowing cognitive functions to reset and the brain to process information more efficiently.

Activities such as meditation, recreational reading, or simply spending time in nature can be effective ways to rest your mind, reducing stress and improving mental clarity.

Furthermore, adequate rest helps maintain emotional balance. People who rest well are better able to manage stress and difficult emotions. Lack of rest, on the other hand, can increase levels of irritability, anxiety, and depression, as the body and mind don't have the time they need to recover from the stresses of everyday life.

This creates a negative cycle in which accumulated stress affects sleep quality, which in turn impacts the ability to cope with emotional challenges, thus worsening overall discomfort. Taking time to rest, both through sleep and conscious pauses throughout the day, is essential for maintaining stable emotional health and improving resilience in the face of life's difficulties.

Physical rest, beyond sleep, is also vital for well-being. After physical exercise or intense activity, the body needs time to recover and heal. Muscles, joints, and connective tissues repair any damage and strengthen during rest.

This recovery process is essential for avoiding injuries, improving physical performance, and maintaining long-term flexibility and endurance. Those who exercise regularly should make sure to incorporate rest periods into their routine, as overtraining can lead to chronic fatigue, decreased immune function, and an increased risk of injury.

In many cultures, rest is considered a central component of overall well-being. In Blue Zones, where people live longer and healthier lives, adequate rest has been observed to be a common practice.

In Ikaria, Greece, for example, it's common for people to take naps during the day, which allows them to regain energy and reduce stress. This custom is associated with a lower incidence of heart disease and better mental health. Similarly, in Loma Linda,

Mindful rest is also a powerful tool for improving productivity and creativity. Regular breaks throughout the day, even just a few minutes, can help prevent mental fatigue and improve performance on cognitive tasks. Often, the best ideas emerge during moments of rest or when disconnected from a particular task. This is because, during rest, the brain continues to subconsciously process information, which facilitates problem-solving and the generation of new ideas.

Ultimately, adequate rest is a cornerstone of overall well-being, affecting all areas of health: physical, mental, and emotional.

From deep sleep that regenerates the body to daily breaks that allow the mind to rest, rest is an active restorative process that improves the ability to face daily challenges and promotes a more balanced and healthy life. Incorporating rest as a fundamental part of your lifestyle is essential for living a fulfilling life with more energy, better health, and greater overall well-being.

Chapter 3.
How to Live Longer and Better: Lessons from the Blue Zones

How to Live Longer and Better: Lessons from the Blue Zones explores the longevity secrets of the world's healthiest and longest-living communities, known as Blue Zones. These areas, spread across regions as diverse as Ikaria in Greece, Okinawa in Japan, Nicoya in Costa Rica, Sardinia in Italy, and Loma Linda in the United States, are examples of how lifestyle and daily habits significantly influence longevity and quality of life.

Based on scientific studies and observations, these communities offer valuable lessons on how to live longer and better, which can be applied in any context, regardless of geographic location.

One of the most important lessons to be learned from the Blue Zones is the importance of a healthy, plant-based diet. In these regions, people consume diets rich in fruits, vegetables, legumes, and whole grains, with very little meat and processed foods.

Plant-based foods, which are rich in antioxidants, fiber, and essential nutrients, contribute to better heart health, a more efficient metabolism, and a reduced risk of chronic diseases such as cancer and diabetes.

In Okinawa, for example, tofu, fish, and purple sweet potatoes are staple foods that have been shown to be effective in prolonging life. Moderation is also key in these communities, where calorie restriction is practiced and people eat until they are approximately 80% full, a custom known as "hara hachi bu" in Okinawa.

Another key lesson is moderate, consistent exercise, which in Blue Zones is part of everyday life rather than a separate activity. People in these regions don't necessarily engage in intense workouts in gyms, but rather integrate movement into their daily routines through activities such as walking, gardening, or household chores.

This regular, but not strenuous, physical activity strengthens the heart, muscles, and bones, and also improves mental health by reducing stress and anxiety.

In Sardinia, Sardinian shepherds walk long distances through mountainous terrain, which helps them stay active and healthy throughout their lives.

A sense of community is another fundamental pillar in the Blue Zones. Deep interpersonal relationships and social support play a crucial role in emotional well-being and longevity. In all these regions, people live surrounded by family, friends, and neighbors with whom they maintain close and meaningful ties.

These social networks provide a sense of belonging and emotional security, which reduces stress and improves mental health. In Okinawa, "moai," groups of close friends who support each other throughout life, are an example of how personal relationships can be a source of well-being and longevity.

Research has shown that people with strong social connections have a longer life expectancy and are less likely to suffer from stress-related illnesses.

Furthermore, a sense of purpose is a shared characteristic of Blue Zone residents. Having a clear reason for getting up each morning, whether in the form of an "ikigai" in Japan or a "life plan" in Nicoya, Costa Rica, provides them with motivation, resilience, and greater life satisfaction.

This sense of purpose not only helps people stay mentally active and engaged, but it's also associated with greater longevity. Those who feel a sense of purpose tend to be more proactive in taking care of their health and are better able to overcome emotional and physical challenges.

Stress management is also a fundamental lesson to be learned from the Blue Zones. Chronic stress is a contributing factor to premature aging and a variety of health problems. In these long-lived regions, people adopt regular practices that allow them to relax and disconnect from daily stresses.

In Icaria, Greece, for example, it's common for people to take daily naps, which helps reduce stress and improve cardiovascular function. In Loma Linda, Seventh-day Adventists observe the Sabbath, a full day of rest dedicated to reflection, prayer, and community, which contributes to their overall well-being.

Finally, Blue Zones also teach the importance of living in balance with nature. In these communities, people often grow their own food, which not only ensures they consume fresh and nutritious produce but also allows them to stay connected to the natural environment. Regular contact with nature has multiple health benefits, including stress reduction, improved mood, and a stronger immune system.

Healthy habits in your daily routine.

Healthy habits in your daily routine. They are the foundation of a full, balanced, and long life. Incorporating simple yet consistent practices into your daily life can significantly transform your physical, mental, and emotional health over time.

Often, these habits don't require great efforts or radical changes, but rather a series of small actions that, when repeated regularly, promote well-being and prevent disease. People who live in Blue Zones, areas of the world where exceptional longevity is achieved, are a clear example of how everyday habits have a profound impact on health.

One of the fundamental pillars of healthy habits is a balanced diet.

Most long-lived individuals adopt a diet rich in natural, minimally processed foods, prioritizing fruits, vegetables, legumes, and whole grains. These foods not only provide the essential nutrients the body needs but are also rich in antioxidants and fiber, which helps reduce the risk of chronic diseases such as diabetes, cancer, and heart disease.

Incorporating fresh, seasonal foods into your daily diet, reducing your consumption of ultra-processed foods, and limiting sugar and saturated fats are simple changes that can have a significant impact on your long-term health.

Furthermore, as we mentioned before, moderation is key; learning to eat until you feel satisfied, but not overly full, as they do in Okinawa with the practice of "hara hachi bu," is an effective strategy for controlling weight and avoiding digestive stress.

Another essential habit is regular physical activity. Staying active doesn't necessarily mean intense workouts or long sessions at the gym. Instead, moderate physical activities, such as walking, cycling, housework, or gardening, can be equally beneficial if done consistently.

Daily physical activity helps keep your heart healthy, strengthens muscles and bones, improves flexibility, and regulates metabolism. Exercise also has positive effects on mental health, reducing stress levels, improving mood, and combating depression.

Residents of Blue Zones, such as the Sardinian shepherds in Sardinia, Italy, exemplify how regular movement through everyday activities is a powerful tool for living longer and better lives.

Adequate rest is also a fundamental component of a healthy routine. Sleeping between seven and nine hours a night allows the body and mind to regenerate, which is crucial for overall well-being. Quality sleep not only helps repair tissues and strengthen the immune system, but also improves cognitive functions, such as memory and decision-making.

People who get adequate rest have more energy during the day, are more productive, and experience fewer mental health problems. In addition to nighttime sleep, taking short breaks during the workday, practicing meditation, or simply disconnecting from screens also helps reduce mental fatigue and improve performance.

Stress management is another key aspect of adopting healthy habits. Chronic stress is one of the major contributing factors to the development of physical and mental illness.

Developing stress management strategies, such as meditation, deep breathing, yoga, or simply dedicating time to hobbies and pleasurable activities, is essential for maintaining emotional balance and reducing tension in the body. In Ikaria, Greece, a relaxed lifestyle and regular naps are examples of how slowing down the daily pace can have positive effects on health.

Interpersonal relationships play an important role in health and well-being. People with strong social relationships tend to be happier, have fewer mental health problems, and enjoy longer lives.

Maintaining connections with friends, family, and colleagues fosters emotional support, reduces loneliness, and provides a safety net during difficult times. Simply making time to interact with others, whether in person or through technology, is a habit that promotes emotional well-being and contributes to longevity.

In Okinawa, Japan, moai is a cultural practice that encourages the creation of close, lifelong support groups, which has been key to their longevity and well-being.

Finally, a sense of purpose is a mental habit that shouldn't be underestimated. Having a clear reason for getting up each day—whether it's a personal project, caring for a family, or contributing to the community—offers powerful motivation to stay active and engaged in life. People with a sense of purpose tend to experience less stress and are more resilient in the face of adversity.

In Nicoya, Costa Rica, the idea of a "life plan" is a reflection of how purpose drives a fuller, more satisfying life.

In conclusion, adopting healthy habits into your daily routine is an effective strategy for improving your quality of life and increasing your longevity. Small changes—such as eating a more balanced diet, exercising regularly, getting adequate rest, managing stress, maintaining meaningful relationships, and having a clear sense of purpose—can make a big difference in your overall health.

These lessons, drawn from the world's longest-living communities, demonstrate that well-being is not achieved through major transformations, but through consistent daily habits that promote physical, mental, and emotional balance.

Stress reduction and its effects on prolonged life.

Stress reduction. It plays a fundamental role in promoting a long and healthy life, as chronic stress is one of the main factors contributing to physical and mental deterioration. Although stress is a natural response of the body to challenges or threats, when prolonged over time without proper management, it can have devastating effects on health.

Research shows that prolonged stress is linked to a higher incidence of cardiovascular disease, hypertension, diabetes, depression, and a weakened immune system. Therefore, learning to manage and reduce stress is essential for those seeking not only to live longer, but also to do so with a better quality of life.

Chronic stress triggers a constant response in the sympathetic nervous system, leading to the release of hormones such as cortisol and adrenaline. While these hormones are helpful in short-term emergency situations, when released continuously, they can cause significant damage to the body.

Elevated cortisol over long periods contributes to increased blood pressure, abdominal fat accumulation, insulin resistance, and a weakened immune system, which increases the risk of chronic disease. Furthermore, chronic stress affects mental health, causing anxiety, insomnia, exhaustion, and a greater susceptibility to depression.

People living in Blue Zones, areas of the world where longevity is most common, have shown that stress reduction is a key strategy for living longer and healthier. In these regions, residents practice natural and effective ways of managing stress as part of their daily lives.

In Ikaria, Greece, for example, it's common to take daily naps, a custom that not only improves physical rest but also reduces stress and blood pressure levels, contributing to better cardiovascular health. This type of planned rest allows the body to relax and recover from daily stresses, which in the long run helps keep the heart and blood vessels healthy.

Taking a weekly break to relax and reflect is an effective way to reduce accumulated stress and restore energy, which has a positive impact on longevity.

Another key factor in stress reduction is social connection. People who maintain strong ties with family, friends, and their community tend to have lower stress levels and therefore enjoy a longer life expectancy. Interpersonal relationships act as an emotional support network, providing comfort and security during difficult times. Social connections not only promote emotional well-being but also protect against stress-related illnesses.

The practice of meditation and spirituality has also been shown to be an effective way to reduce stress. Meditation, prayer, and other forms of inner reflection allow the mind and body to enter a state of calm, which decreases the release of cortisol and improves emotional health.

Many long-lived individuals attribute their well-being to an active spiritual life, where religious or philosophical beliefs provide them with a sense of purpose and help them find inner peace, even during difficult times.

In Ikaria and Okinawa, spirituality plays a crucial role in people's ability to cope with difficulties without being overwhelmed by stress.

In addition to these strategies, contact with nature is another factor that contributes to stress reduction and, ultimately, a longer life. Spending time outdoors, surrounded by nature, has been shown to have calming effects on the nervous system, lowering blood pressure and promoting a sense of well-being.

In Nicoya, Costa Rica, residents often work their land and spend much of their time outdoors, which not only keeps them physically active but also allows them to enjoy the relaxing benefits of the natural environment. Contact with nature helps reduce stress, improves mood, and provides a sense of connection with one's surroundings, which contributes to greater life satisfaction.

Moderation as a principle of life.

Moderation as a principle of lifeIt is an essential approach to maintaining health, well-being, and longevity. This concept lies at the heart of many life philosophies and cultural traditions that promote balance, contentment, and the prevention of excess.

Moderation involves avoiding extremes—whether in diet, work, leisure, or resource consumption—and seeking a middle ground that achieves harmony in all aspects of life. In Blue Zones, where people live longer and enjoy a better quality of life, moderation is a central pillar of their daily habits.

One of the areas where moderation is most evident and effective is in nutrition. Instead of consuming large amounts of food or binge eating, people who practice moderation focus on smaller, balanced portions, which contributes to better digestion and a healthier life.

This habit prevents excess calories and helps maintain a healthy weight, reducing the risk of obesity and associated chronic diseases, such as diabetes and cardiovascular problems. This practice of moderation also boosts metabolism and contributes to greater longevity.

Dietary moderation also involves choosing foods that are natural, fresh, and nutrient-dense, but without resorting to deprivation or strict diets. In the Blue Zones, plant-based diets, which include a variety of fruits, vegetables, legumes, and whole grains, are an example of how moderation can be applied to food selection.

These people consume meat and processed foods only in small amounts or on special occasions, allowing them to maintain a nutrient-dense diet without the risks associated with overconsuming unhealthy foods. This moderate approach is not only beneficial for the body but also fosters a more conscious and balanced relationship with food.

In addition to nutrition, moderation at work is crucial for maintaining a healthy lifestyle. Stress related to overwork is one of the factors that most negatively affects physical and mental health in modern society.

People who don't practice moderation in their work lives often face burnout, anxiety, and health problems such as high blood pressure or heart disease. In Blue Zones, however, work is balanced with rest and leisure.

The inhabitants of Icaria, Greece, and Nicoya, Costa Rica, for example, practice a lifestyle where work doesn't dominate their lives, but rather is balanced with moments of relaxation, social interaction, and recreational activities. This moderation in work life allows the body and mind to recover, reducing stress and promoting greater longevity.

The balance between activity and rest is another area where moderation plays a key role. Physical exercise is vital for maintaining good health, but excessive activity can be as harmful as a lack of movement. In Blue Zones, people consistently engage in moderate physical activity, such as walking, housework, or gardening, allowing them to stay active without overtaxing their bodies.

Moderation in exercise helps prevent injuries, improves cardiovascular health, and maintains strong muscles and bones. At the same time, rest is equally valued. Taking time to rest, sleep well, and disconnect from daily obligations is essential for proper recovery and overall well-being.

Moderation in resource consumption is also a principle that contributes to sustainability and a balanced lifestyle. Instead of consuming recklessly and without considering the long-term impact, people who practice moderation adopt a more conscious and responsible approach to resource use.

This not only has environmental benefits but also reduces the financial stress and anxiety associated with consumerism. In Blue Zones, people tend to live more simply and self-sufficiently, growing their own food and sharing resources with the community, allowing them to enjoy a full life without indulging in material excess.

Emotional balance is another fundamental aspect of moderation as a life principle. People who practice emotional moderation know how to manage their emotions without being dominated by them.

They don't get carried away by excessive anger, anxiety, or sadness, nor do they repress their emotions to the point of feeling disconnected. Instead of oscillating between emotional extremes, moderate people maintain a calm and balanced approach to life's challenges.

This emotional control is key to mental well-being and maintaining healthy relationships with others.

Finally, moderation in the pace of life is essential to achieving comprehensive well-being. We live in an era where everything seems to move at breakneck speed, generating constant stress. People who adopt a moderate approach to life know how to slow down, enjoy the present, and avoid the burnout caused by a fast-paced lifestyle.

In Blue Zones, people value time to relax, spend time with family and friends, and enjoy simple activities such as conversation, a shared meal, or a walk outdoors. This calmer, more balanced pace of life not only reduces stress but also promotes a longer, healthier life.

The relationship between life purpose and longevity.

The relationship between life purpose and longevity is a link that has been studied in various scientific studies, and it has been shown that having a clear sense of purpose can have a significant impact on the length and quality of life.

Life purpose refers to a personal, deep, and meaningful reason for living, which gives direction and meaning to daily actions.

This sense of purpose acts as a constant source of motivation that helps people stay active, resilient, and engaged with their environment, which has positive effects on physical, mental, and emotional health.

In the Blue Zones, where people have extraordinary life expectancies, life purpose is a common factor contributing to their longevity. In Okinawa, Japan, residents refer to this concept as "ikigai," which literally means "the reason for getting up in the morning." For Okinawans, having ikigai is crucial to maintaining an active and healthy life.

Whether it's caring for their family, participating in the community, or committing to a personal project, this purpose drives them to continue, even into advanced age. In Nicoya, Costa Rica, the term "life plan" is used to describe the purpose that guides people's existence and provides them with a stable emotional foundation that, according to studies, contributes to greater longevity.

Life purpose has a direct impact on longevity because it influences several key areas of well-being. First, people with a strong sense of purpose tend to have better physical health. By having a clear reason for living, these people often take better care of their bodies and make healthier choices throughout their lives.

They are more likely to maintain a balanced diet, exercise regularly, and avoid harmful habits such as excessive alcohol consumption or tobacco. Furthermore, purpose motivates them to stay physically and mentally active, which promotes heart health, strengthens muscles, and maintains mental sharpness.

From an emotional perspective, life purpose helps people better cope with challenges and adversity. Those who feel their lives have a deeper meaning are more resilient in the face of stress and difficulties, which reduces the negative impact of chronic stress on their health.

Prolonged stress is known to be a major factor in the development of diseases such as hypertension, heart problems, and immune disorders. However, people with a strong sense of purpose have a greater ability to adapt to difficult situations, allowing them to manage stress more effectively and protect their health. This sense of resilience also promotes emotional stability, which contributes to a more balanced and fulfilling life.

In social terms, people with a life purpose tend to establish and maintain more meaningful and deeper relationships. Purpose not only drives them to act in their own best interest, but is often linked to a desire to contribute to others and the community. This sense of contribution strengthens social ties, which has positive effects on mental and emotional health.

Close social connections, such as those seen in Blue Zones, not only provide emotional support, but also contribute to greater life satisfaction and a reduction in loneliness and isolation, factors that are often linked to higher mortality.

Furthermore, life purpose is linked to long-term cognitive health. People who find meaning in their lives and stay mentally active are less likely to develop neurodegenerative diseases such as Alzheimer's or dementia.

Constant engagement with a meaningful task—whether intellectual, social, or physical—keeps the brain active and stimulated, which protects cognitive function. This protective effect of life purpose on mental and cognitive health is a key reason why many long-lived individuals in the Blue Zones manage to remain mentally agile and have good memories even in old age.

The impact of life purpose is not limited to the physical and emotional aspects. Spirituality also plays an important role in how life purpose influences longevity. Many people find their purpose through faith or spirituality, which provides them with a solid foundation of beliefs that helps them cope with suffering and uncertainty.

Having a transcendental perspective on life and death can reduce fear of mortality and provide a sense of inner peace that contributes to a longer, more balanced life.

Finally, life purpose provides an intrinsic motivation to continue learning and growing, even in later life. People who feel they have a clear purpose tend to adopt a growth mindset, where they are open to new experiences and willing to continue developing personally and professionally.

This approach not only improves quality of life but also contributes to maintaining curiosity and enthusiasm for life, two factors that have been associated with greater longevity.

Chapter 4.
Lifestyle Habits That Increase Your Life Expectancy

The lifestyle habits that increase your life expectancy are directly related to daily practices that promote physical, mental, and emotional health over time. These habits, when consistently integrated into your daily routine, can make a significant difference in longevity and quality of life.

In the Blue Zones, where people enjoy longer and healthier lives, several key habits have been identified that contribute to a longer life expectancy. These habits don't require drastic changes, but rather sustainable adjustments that can be adopted by anyone, anywhere in the world.

One of the most important habits for increasing life expectancy is maintaining a balanced, plant-based diet. Research has shown that a diet rich in fruits, vegetables, legumes, whole grains, and nuts is associated with a lower incidence of chronic diseases, such as heart disease, diabetes, and cancer.

People who follow a predominantly plant-based diet consume foods packed with nutrients, antioxidants, and fiber, which help protect the body from cellular damage and promote healthy digestion. In Blue Zones, such as Okinawa, Japan, and Nicoya, Costa Rica, people eat moderate portions of fresh, local foods, with limited consumption of meat and processed products.

Regular, moderate exercise is another key habit for increasing life expectancy. Unlike modern societies, where exercise is often seen as a structured activity in a gym, in Blue Zones people stay active naturally throughout the day.

Walking, biking, gardening, or doing housework are forms of consistent movement that not only strengthen the body but also improve cardiovascular health and maintain mobility for years to come. Moderate physical activity reduces the risk of obesity, heart disease, and diabetes, while also improving mood and reducing stress. Staying active regularly not only helps prolong life but also improves the quality of that life by maintaining independence and functional ability as we age.

Stress management is another essential component of lifestyle habits that promote longevity. Chronic stress is linked to a wide variety of health problems, ranging from cardiovascular disease to immune system disorders.

Learning to manage stress through practices such as meditation, deep breathing, yoga, or simply taking regular breaks is crucial to keeping the body and mind balanced. In Ikaria, Greece, for example, people enjoy a peaceful life where daily naps are common, which helps reduce blood pressure and improve cardiovascular health.

In Loma Linda, California, Seventh-day Adventists dedicate a full day each week to rest and spiritual reflection, helping them disconnect from stress and focus on their personal well-being.

Adequate rest, particularly restorative sleep, is a habit that should not be underestimated for its impact on longevity. Sleeping between seven and nine hours a night allows the body and mind to regenerate, which is vital for overall health.

During sleep, the body repairs tissues, strengthens the immune system, and balances hormones that control stress and hunger. Lack of adequate sleep has been linked to an increased risk of chronic diseases such as diabetes and hypertension, as well as decreased cognitive function.

Therefore, establishing a healthy sleep routine and prioritizing adequate rest is a habit that can significantly prolong life.

Strong social relationships are also a crucial factor for longevity. People who maintain deep connections with family, friends, and their community have lower stress levels and greater life satisfaction. These social connections provide emotional support, help reduce feelings of loneliness and isolation, and promote a sense of belonging.

In Okinawa, the concept of "moai" brings together groups of close friends who support each other throughout life, providing a consistent supportive environment that strengthens emotional health. Research suggests that people with strong social networks not only live longer but also have a better quality of life, with fewer mental and emotional health problems.

A sense of purpose is another key habit that contributes to a longer life expectancy. Having a clear reason for getting up each morning, whether it's a personal project, caring for a family, or participating in the community, provides direction and motivation for daily life.

Purpose not only keeps people mentally active and engaged, but also promotes a positive attitude toward aging and greater life satisfaction.

Finally, moderation in all areas of life is an essential principle for increasing longevity. In the Blue Zones, people practice moderation not only in their diet, but also in their approach to work, exercise, and resource consumption.

Avoiding excesses and maintaining balance in all aspects of life reduces the risk of stress-related illnesses and burnout. Moderation allows people to enjoy life without resorting to extremes that can harm their long-term health.

The importance of light but constant physical activity.

Light but consistent physical activity is one of the fundamental pillars for maintaining good health and prolonging life. Unlike the intensive workouts and exhausting routines often associated with exercise, light physical activity, performed consistently throughout the day, offers equally powerful benefits for physical, mental, and emotional well-being.

This approach, seen in many Blue Zones, where people reach advanced age with vitality and health, demonstrates that strenuous exercise isn't necessary to live longer. Rather, it's consistency in daily movement that makes the difference.

Light physical activity refers to everyday movements such as walking, climbing stairs, gardening, cycling, cleaning the house, or any other activity that keeps the body moving smoothly and continuously.

This type of exercise is easily integrated into a daily routine, making it sustainable over the long term. Rather than requiring dedicated gym sessions, people who practice light physical activity naturally incorporate it into their lifestyles. In Blue Zones, such as Sardinia, Italy, and Okinawa, Japan, it's common to see older adults walking long distances, tending to their gardens, or performing household chores without considering them "exercise" in the conventional sense, yet these activities are key to their longevity.

One of the most important benefits of regular physical activity is its impact on cardiovascular health. Light, yet regular, movement stimulates blood circulation, strengthens the heart, and helps maintain healthy blood pressure.

People who are consistently physically active throughout the day have a lower risk of developing heart disease, as their hearts become stronger and can pump blood more efficiently. Furthermore, this type of activity helps regulate blood cholesterol levels, reducing the risk of arterial blockages and, therefore, heart attacks or strokes.

Light physical activity is also extremely beneficial for weight management and metabolic health. Although light exercise doesn't burn as many calories at once as high-intensity exercise, its steady-state nature helps maintain an active metabolism throughout the day.

This helps prevent weight gain and the accumulation of abdominal fat, factors that are linked to an increased risk of metabolic diseases such as type 2 diabetes. By moving regularly, the body also uses insulin better, which helps regulate blood sugar levels and prevent spikes and drops that can affect energy and overall well-being.

Another key aspect of light, consistent physical activity is its contribution to muscle and bone health. Over the years, it's common for people to experience a gradual loss of muscle mass and bone density, which can lead to problems such as osteoporosis or loss of mobility.

However, staying active with light exercise, such as walking or performing everyday tasks, helps preserve muscle strength and flexibility. This type of gentle movement also stimulates bone cell production, which helps keep bones strong and reduces the risk of fractures.

People who engage in light but consistent physical activity are more likely to remain agile and mobile even in old age, enabling them to lead independent and fulfilling lives.

In terms of mental health, consistent physical activity also plays a crucial role. Regular movement helps release endorphins, hormones that improve mood and reduce stress. People who stay active tend to experience less anxiety and depression, as exercise acts as a natural mood regulator.

In addition, light exercise promotes mental clarity and concentration, as it increases blood flow to the brain and stimulates cognitive function. This is especially important in older age, as regular physical activity has been shown to be an effective tool for preventing cognitive decline and neurodegenerative diseases such as Alzheimer's.

Regular physical activity is also essential for sleep regulation. People who move regularly throughout the day tend to have better quality sleep at night. Light exercise helps regulate the body's circadian rhythms, making it easier to fall asleep and enjoy deeper, more restful sleep.

Adequate sleep, in turn, is essential for cell regeneration, memory consolidation, and hormonal balance. Those who stay active during the day are less likely to suffer from insomnia or sleep disruptions, allowing them to wake up with more energy and vitality.

Furthermore, light physical activity is accessible to people of all ages and physical conditions, making it an ideal option for those looking to improve their health without the risks associated with high-intensity exercise. Walking, for example, is an activity that almost anyone can do, and its positive impact on health is undeniable.

In Blue Zones, older adults continue to stay physically active through daily walks and other gentle activities, allowing them to maintain their mobility and independence far beyond what is common in other parts of the world.

Balanced nutrition: key foods for a long life.

A balanced diet is essential for a long and healthy life, as it provides the essential nutrients the body needs to function optimally and prevent chronic diseases.

In the Blue Zones, where people live longer and with better quality of life, diet plays a central role in their longevity. These communities, located in regions such as Okinawa (Japan), Nicoya (Costa Rica), Icaria (Greece), Sardinia (Italy), and Loma Linda (United States), have adopted dietary practices that promote health and well-being throughout life.

The key foods they consume are natural, nutrient-dense, and low in saturated fats and processed foods, which contributes to reducing the risk of disease and promoting a longer life.

One of the most important components of a balanced diet is the consumption of fresh fruits and vegetables. These foods are rich in vitamins, minerals, antioxidants, and fiber, all of which are essential for maintaining body health and protecting it from cell damage.

Fruits and vegetables are particularly rich in antioxidants, which help combat oxidative stress and reduce inflammation, key factors that contribute to aging and the development of chronic diseases such as cancer and heart disease.

In the Blue Zones, residents consume a wide variety of local and seasonal produce, such as broccoli, carrots, tomatoes, spinach, and sweet potatoes, which form the basis of their diets. These foods not only provide a wealth of essential nutrients but are also low in calories, helping to maintain a healthy weight and prevent obesity, another major risk factor for long-term health.

Another essential group for a balanced diet is legumes. Foods such as beans, lentils, chickpeas, and peas are an important source of plant-based protein, fiber, and micronutrients. Legumes are not only rich in protein but also low in fat and cholesterol-free, making them an ideal choice for those looking to reduce their risk of heart disease.

In addition, its high fiber content helps improve digestion and maintain stable blood sugar levels, which is crucial for preventing type 2 diabetes.

In Nicoya, Costa Rica, black beans are a daily staple, while in Icaria and Sardinia, lentils and chickpeas are part of many traditional meals. These staples are nutritious, affordable, and filling, contributing to a balanced diet that promotes longevity.

Healthy fats also play a crucial role in a diet that promotes a long life. In the Blue Zones, fat consumption comes primarily from plant sources such as olive oil and nuts, rather than animal fats or ultra-processed products.

Olive oil, particularly in Icaria and Sardinia, is an important source of monounsaturated fats, which have been shown to protect the heart and reduce LDL ("bad") cholesterol levels.

These healthy fats also have anti-inflammatory properties that help keep blood vessels flexible and prevent plaque buildup in the arteries, reducing the risk of cardiovascular disease. Nuts, such as almonds and walnuts, which are common in the Loma Linda diet, are rich in omega-3 fatty acids, which also support heart health and protect the brain against cognitive decline.

Whole grains are another essential component of a balanced diet and long life. Unlike refined grains, whole grains like oats, brown rice, quinoa, and whole wheat retain their natural fiber and essential nutrients, making them a much healthier choice.

Whole grains are an excellent source of slow-release energy, which helps maintain stable blood glucose levels and prevent insulin spikes. This is especially important for preventing metabolic diseases like type 2 diabetes.

In Okinawa, brown rice and purple sweet potatoes are staple foods that provide long-lasting energy and are packed with nutrients that support gut and cardiovascular health. In Nicoya, whole-grain corn is also a key source of complex carbohydrates that support daily energy.

Plant-based protein, such as that from legumes, grains, and nuts, is another key element in longevity. Instead of relying on large amounts of red or processed meat, which has been linked to an increased risk of cancer and heart disease, long-lived people in Blue Zones get most of their protein from plant sources.

These proteins are not only easier to digest, but also contain less saturated fat and calories, which helps maintain a healthy weight and reduces the risk of diet-related diseases. In Sardinia, for example, sheep's milk cheese is a source of protein consumed in moderation, while in Okinawa, tofu is a staple food that provides complete protein without the risks associated with processed meat.

Another key aspect of balanced nutrition in the Blue Zones is moderation in food consumption. Residents of these regions tend to eat smaller portions and avoid overindulging. In Okinawa, the practice of "hara hachi bu" teaches people to stop eating when they are 80% full, which helps avoid calorie overload and reduces stress on the digestive system.

This moderation is also observed in limited alcohol consumption. In Blue Zones, people who drink do so in moderation, usually in the form of red wine with meals, which has been shown to have positive effects on cardiovascular health thanks to its antioxidant content, such as resveratrol.

In conclusion, a balanced diet rich in fruits, vegetables, legumes, whole grains, healthy fats, and plant-based proteins is key to a long and healthy life. Natural, minimally processed foods provide the body with the essential nutrients it needs to function optimally, while moderation in food consumption helps maintain calorie balance and prevents the development of chronic diseases.

The lessons of the Blue Zones show us that eating well is not just about what foods we eat, but how we integrate them into our daily lives, maintaining a balanced and moderate diet that promotes longevity and long-term well-being.

Healthy personal relationships as a pillar of well-being.

Healthy personal relationships are one of the fundamental pillars of well-being and have a profound impact on quality of life and longevity. Several studies have shown that people who maintain strong, positive social ties enjoy better physical and mental health, experience less stress, and are better able to cope with life's challenges.

In Blue Zones, areas of the world where people reach advanced ages with a remarkable quality of life, interpersonal relationships play a crucial role in their longevity. These communities value emotional support, family connections, and a sense of belonging, which helps them live healthier and happier lives.

One of the main reasons healthy relationships are so important for well-being is their ability to reduce stress. Chronic stress is linked to a number of serious health problems, including heart disease, hypertension, and immune system disorders.

However, people who have an emotional support network, whether through family, friends, or colleagues, tend to handle stress better. These relationships act as an emotional safety net, providing comfort and relief in times of difficulty.

Sharing problems and concerns with loved ones not only reduces the emotional burden but also allows situations to be viewed from different perspectives, facilitating decision-making and problem-solving.

In communities like Okinawa, Japan, "moai," small groups of friends who support each other throughout life, provide a strong support system that helps reduce stress and promote longevity.

In addition to stress management, healthy personal relationships have a direct impact on physical health. People who maintain close and meaningful connections tend to adopt healthier behaviors. Social support encourages positive lifestyle habits, such as exercising, maintaining a balanced diet, and avoiding risky behaviors like smoking or excessive alcohol consumption.

For example, in Blue Zones, it's common for people to gather to share healthy meals, engage in light physical activity, and participate in community events, reinforcing their healthy habits and keeping them active. Studies have also shown that social isolation and loneliness increase the risk of cardiovascular disease, while people with strong social networks are more likely to live longer and healthier lives.

Interpersonal relationships are also essential for mental well-being. The sense of belonging to a community and being connected to others improves mood, reduces anxiety levels, and prevents depression.

In Loma Linda, California, one of the Blue Zones, Seventh-day Adventists not only support one another through faith and community activities, but also benefit from intergenerational relationships, where elders and youth interact regularly, fostering a sense of purpose and belonging at all stages of life.

This intergenerational interaction also provides a valuable emotional support network that is critical to mental well-being.

Another crucial aspect of healthy relationships is their ability to foster a sense of purpose. Being connected to others and feeling part of something bigger can give deep meaning to daily life.

In Nicoya, Costa Rica, older adults often have a "life plan," a clear reason for getting up each morning, whether to care for their families, participate in the community, or maintain active social relationships. This sense of purpose not only improves emotional well-being but is also linked to increased longevity.

People who feel meaningful in their lives tend to be more active, resilient, and optimistic, which contributes to better physical and mental health.

Furthermore, healthy personal relationships are key to developing emotional resilience in the face of life's challenges. People who have a close support network tend to be better able to overcome difficulties, as they feel supported and supported during difficult times.

Emotional resilience not only helps manage stress and negative emotions, but also allows for faster and more effective recovery after adverse situations. Healthy relationships provide a solid emotional foundation that acts as a buffer against the negative effects of chronic stress and life's difficulties.

Another important benefit of healthy relationships is the cognitive stimulation they provide.

Regular social interactions, such as conversation, discussion, and sharing experiences, keep the brain active and engaged, which is essential for preventing cognitive decline and neurodegenerative diseases.

People who maintain meaningful interpersonal relationships tend to be more mentally agile and less likely to develop dementia or Alzheimer's.

In Blue Zones, it is common for older adults to remain actively involved in community conversations and activities, which contributes to their longevity and long-term mental health.

Finally, healthy personal relationships also influence overall well-being by providing a sense of belonging and emotional security.

Knowing that you have the support of loved ones and a community not only reduces feelings of loneliness but also increases self-esteem and a sense of personal worth. People who feel loved and valued tend to have a more positive attitude toward life and face challenges with greater optimism.

This sense of belonging is also associated with a lower incidence of mental health problems and greater overall life satisfaction.

Healthy personal relationships are a fundamental pillar of well-being and longevity. These connections not only reduce stress and improve physical health, but also strengthen mental well-being, promote healthy habits, and provide a sense of purpose and belonging.

The lessons of the Blue Zones show that emotional support and meaningful relationships not only contribute to a longer life, but also significantly improve the quality of that life, demonstrating that the true wealth of well-being lies in deep, healthy human connections.

Techniques to maintain a positive mindset over the years.

Maintaining a positive mindset over the years is essential to enjoying a full, balanced life with emotional well-being. A positive mindset not only influences how we perceive and face daily challenges, but also has a significant impact on our physical and mental health.

As we age, it's crucial to develop strategies that allow us to maintain a positive, resilient, and open attitude toward continuous learning, as this can contribute to a higher quality of life and even greater longevity.

There are various techniques that can help us cultivate and maintain a positive mindset over the years, based on self-awareness, thought control, stress management, and strengthening interpersonal relationships.

One of the most effective techniques for maintaining a positive mindset is the practice of daily gratitude. Gratitude involves focusing our attention on the positive aspects of life, recognizing and appreciating what we have instead of focusing on what we lack. This approach not only helps us feel more fulfilled and happy, but also reduces stress and improves mental health.

Practicing gratitude can be as simple as keeping a journal where you write down three things you're grateful for each day, or taking a few minutes at the end of the day to reflect on positive moments.

Over time, this practice strengthens our ability to see the bright side of situations and maintain a more optimistic attitude toward life's challenges.

Another key technique is self-awareness. Over the years, it's essential to become aware of our thought patterns and recognize when we're slipping into negative or self-destructive thoughts.

Self-reflection allows us to identify limiting beliefs or cognitive distortions, such as overgeneralization or personalization of negative events. Developing a positive mindset involves changing these negative thinking patterns for more realistic and constructive approaches.

For example, instead of thinking "I never achieve what I set out to do," we can reframe it as "I've had challenges, but I continue to learn and improve with each experience." This cognitive restructuring is a powerful technique for transforming the way we interpret the events in our lives, helping us see opportunities where we previously saw only obstacles.

Stress management is another crucial technique for maintaining a positive mindset over the years. Prolonged stress can negatively affect our outlook on life, making us more prone to pessimism and anxiety.

Learning to manage stress through techniques such as meditation, deep breathing, or mindfulness can help us stay calm and respond more positively to difficult situations. Mindfulness, in particular, is useful for developing greater awareness of the present moment, allowing us to observe our thoughts and emotions without judging them or reacting impulsively.

By practicing mindfulness, we can learn to accept circumstances as they are and reduce emotional reactivity, allowing us to maintain a more balanced and positive perspective.

Proactive optimism is another technique that helps us maintain a positive mindset. Being optimistic doesn't mean ignoring problems or avoiding facing them, but rather trusting that we can find solutions and opportunities for growth amidst difficulties.

Proactive optimism involves taking active steps to improve our situation, rather than getting caught up in worry or fear. Setting realistic and achievable goals and working toward them with perseverance reinforces our sense of accomplishment and increases our self-esteem. This attitude allows us to view challenges as opportunities to learn and improve, rather than as personal failures.

Emotional resilience is another key technique for maintaining a positive mindset over the years. Resilience refers to our ability to adapt and recover from difficulties.

Developing this skill involves accepting that problems are an inevitable part of life, but that we have the power to choose how we react to them. People who practice resilience tend to have a positive attitude because they believe in their ability to overcome obstacles.

To foster resilience, it's helpful to learn to manage emotions constructively, practicing self-care, seeking support from friends or family, and maintaining a balanced perspective in times of crisis.

Another important aspect of maintaining a positive mindset is fostering healthy interpersonal relationships. Positive social connections provide us with emotional support, reduce stress, and help us maintain a more optimistic outlook on life.

Surrounding ourselves with people who encourage us, share our joys, and are there for us during difficult times is crucial to our emotional well-being. Furthermore, the act of giving and receiving support strengthens our self-esteem and reminds us that we are not alone on life's journey.

In Blue Zones, where people live longer and with better quality of life, meaningful personal relationships are a key factor in maintaining a positive and long-lasting mindset.

Physical care also plays an important role in maintaining a positive mindset. Regular exercise, a balanced diet, and adequate rest not only improve our physical health but also have a positive impact on our mental health.

Exercise, for example, releases endorphins, hormones that improve mood and combat stress. Taking care of our bodies makes us feel better about ourselves, which boosts our self-esteem and helps us maintain a more positive attitude.

Finally, continuous learning is an essential technique for maintaining a positive mindset over the years.

Learning new skills, discovering new interests, or simply staying open to new ideas helps us stay mentally sharp and engaged in life.

This approach to constant growth allows us to face aging with an attitude of curiosity and enthusiasm, rather than fear. People who continue to learn and develop are more likely to maintain a positive outlook on life and feel fulfilled as they age.

Chapter 5.
The Path to Healthy and Fulfilling Longevity

The path to healthy and fulfilling longevity is a journey not based solely on genetics, but on the lifestyle habits we cultivate every day. Living longer and in good health is not a destiny reserved for a select few; it is the result of conscious choices that improve our physical, mental, and emotional well-being over time.

People who achieve healthy and fulfilling longevity do so by adopting a balanced lifestyle based on principles such as proper nutrition, regular exercise, stress management, maintaining meaningful relationships, and a clear sense of purpose. These factors not only extend life but also ensure that those additional years are lived with quality, vitality, and satisfaction.

One of the first pillars of the path to healthy longevity is a balanced diet. What we eat has a profound impact on our long-term health.

People who live longer tend to follow a diet rich in natural, minimally processed foods, with a focus on fruits, vegetables, legumes, whole grains, and healthy fats. In regions like the Blue Zones, home to some of the world's longest-lived populations, diet is crucial.

In Okinawa, Japan, for example, eating purple sweet potatoes, tofu, fish, and seaweed provides a wealth of antioxidant and anti-inflammatory nutrients that promote cellular and cardiovascular health. Furthermore, these communities practice moderation in food, with habits such as "hara hachi bu," which involves eating until you are 80% full.

This moderation prevents excess calories, which helps prevent diseases such as obesity and diabetes, which can shorten life expectancy.

The second pillar is consistent but moderate physical activity. Unlike intensive workouts, which are often seen as the only way to stay fit, long-lived people integrate natural movement into their daily lives. Walking, doing housework, gardening, or even caring for animals are all forms of physical activity that keep the body moving without the need for formal training.

This type of daily exercise helps strengthen the heart, improve blood circulation, and maintain mobility as we age. Furthermore, regular physical activity contributes to the prevention of chronic diseases, such as heart disease and type 2 diabetes, and promotes mental health by reducing stress and improving mood.

Effective stress management

Another fundamental aspect of the path to healthy longevity is effective stress management. Chronic stress negatively impacts health, as it can weaken the immune system, increase the risk of heart disease, and cause digestive problems, among other things. Learning to manage stress through techniques such as meditation, deep breathing, yoga, or simply taking regular breaks is key to a long and balanced life.

In Icaria, Greece, for example, daily naps are a custom that helps reduce stress levels, contributing to longevity. Similarly, in Loma Linda, California, Seventh-day Adventists observe a full day of rest and spiritual reflection each week, allowing them to disconnect from everyday stresses and focus on their emotional and physical well-being.

Restful sleep is also crucial on the path to healthy longevity. Sleeping between seven and nine hours a night allows the body to regenerate, strengthens its immune system, and regulates stress hormones. Lack of adequate sleep can increase the risk of chronic diseases, such as diabetes, hypertension, and obesity, and can also negatively affect mood and cognitive function.

Establishing a healthy sleep routine, avoiding the use of electronic devices before bed, and creating a relaxing environment are strategies that promote restful sleep, which is essential for maintaining vitality over the years.

Another key pillar for full longevity is a sense of purpose.

Having a clear reason for getting up every morning—whether it's contributing to the community, taking care of a family, or pursuing a personal project—gives life a meaning that goes beyond everyday tasks. In the Blue Zones, the "ikigai" of Okinawans and the "life plan" of Nicoyans in Costa Rica are examples of how purpose guides longevity.

This sense of purpose not only motivates people to stay active and mentally engaged, but also reduces stress and gives them a reason to keep going, even in later life. People who feel their lives have a purpose experience less depression, have greater emotional resilience, and tend to live longer than those who lack a clear sense of direction.

Maintaining meaningful personal relationships is another essential factor for healthy longevity. The emotional support provided by friends, family, and community has a direct impact on physical and mental health. People who maintain deep social connections tend to have fewer stress-related health problems and are more likely to adopt healthy habits, such as exercising regularly and eating well.

In Okinawa, "moai"—groups of close friends who support each other throughout life—are an example of how social relationships strengthen well-being.

Research shows that people with strong social networks are more likely to live longer and with better quality of life, as social interactions not only reduce the risk of loneliness and depression but also foster a sense of belonging and emotional security.

A positive mindset is also an essential pillar for fulfilling longevity. Throughout life, it's natural to face difficulties and challenges, but how we react to them directly influences our health and well-being.

Cultivate a positive mindset

People who cultivate a positive mindset, which includes gratitude, optimism, and the ability to find the silver lining in situations, tend to be more resilient and live longer. Optimism doesn't mean ignoring problems, but rather facing them with a proactive attitude, trusting in the ability to overcome and learn from them. This mindset contributes to better mental health, less stress, and greater life satisfaction.

In short, the path to healthy and fulfilling longevity is not just about living longer, but about enjoying those years with good health, vitality, and purpose. A balanced diet, consistent physical activity, stress management, adequate rest, meaningful personal relationships, and a clear sense of purpose are the pillars that support this journey toward a long and fulfilling life.

Consciously and consistently adopting these habits can not only increase longevity, but also ensure that those additional years are lived to the fullest, with physical, emotional, and mental well-being.

The lessons learned from long-lived individuals in the Blue Zones show us that longevity is not just a matter of genetics, but of daily choices that promote a life rich in health, happiness, and meaning.

How the natural environment influences health.

The natural environment profoundly influences people's physical, mental, and emotional health. The relationship between humans and their environment has been extensively studied, and findings reveal that natural spaces, such as parks, forests, mountains, beaches, and gardens, have a positive impact on quality of life and overall well-being.

As the world becomes increasingly urbanized, access to nature has become critical for maintaining a healthy balance.

Being in contact with nature not only reduces stress and improves mood, but also strengthens the immune system, promotes physical activity, and contributes to greater longevity.

One of the main benefits of living or spending time in nature is its ability to reduce stress. The fast-paced nature of modern life, work demands, traffic, and constant exposure to technology can increase stress levels, which has negative effects on health.

However, studies have shown that simply being in contact with nature, such as walking in a park or being near a body of water, decreases the production of cortisol, the stress hormone. This relaxing effect of nature helps lower blood pressure, reduce anxiety, and improve sleep quality.

The practice of "shinrin-yoku," or "forest bathing," in Japan is an example of how cultures have integrated the natural environment into their daily well-being. Walking slowly through a forest, breathing in the fresh air and connecting with one's surroundings, has been shown to be an effective tool for reducing stress and improving mental health.

In addition to reducing stress, a natural environment promotes physical activity, which is essential for physical and mental health. People who live near green areas or parks are more likely to walk, run, cycle, or play outdoor sports. Regular physical activity not only improves cardiovascular health and strengthens muscles and bones, but also helps maintain a healthy weight and prevent chronic diseases such as type 2 diabetes and hypertension.

Natural environments also encourage recreational activities, such as gardening, hiking, or outdoor yoga, which not only benefit the body but also contribute to relaxation and emotional well-being.

In Blue Zones, where people live longer, communities are located in natural environments that facilitate regular physical activity, such as in Sardinia, where residents walk in hills and mountains every day as part of their normal routine.

The natural environment also has a direct impact on mental health. Spending time in nature improves mood, reduces depression, and fosters a greater sense of overall well-being.

Research suggests that people who spend more time outdoors have lower anxiety levels and higher levels of life satisfaction.

This is due, in part, to nature's ability to disconnect people from everyday worries and provide a sense of calm and perspective. Contact with nature also improves cognitive function, allowing the mind to rest and recover from mental fatigue.

People who have access to natural environments tend to be more creative, have better concentration, and are more productive in their daily activities. Furthermore, natural surroundings positively stimulate the senses, offering a rich variety of sounds, colors, and textures that are pleasing to the brain.

Another key aspect is that exposure to natural light has a significant impact on the regulation of circadian rhythms, which control sleep-wake cycles. Spending time outdoors and receiving sufficient sunlight during the day helps regulate the production of melatonin, the hormone that facilitates sleep.

A lack of natural light, especially indoors or during winter in colder regions, can cause sleep disturbances and increase the risk of seasonal depression. Moderate sun exposure is also crucial for the production of vitamin D, which is essential for bone health and the immune system. People who spend time in nature tend to have higher levels of vitamin D, which protects them against diseases like osteoporosis and improves their resistance to infections.

The natural environment also has a restorative effect.

The natural environment also has a restorative effect on the immune system. Plants and trees release volatile organic compounds that, when inhaled, stimulate the production of NK (natural killer) cells, which are responsible for fighting viruses and tumors.

This exposure to phytoncides present in forests is one of the reasons why forest bathing not only reduces stress but also strengthens the body's defenses. Furthermore, the fresh air and less pollution in natural areas allow for better oxygenation of the lungs, which improves respiratory capacity and reduces the risk of respiratory diseases.

Another benefit of the natural environment is its ability to foster a sense of connection and belonging. People who spend time in nature often report feeling a deeper connection to the world around them, which promotes greater gratitude and a sense of inner peace.

This connection also reinforces a sense of responsibility toward environmental preservation and the well-being of future generations. In many cultures, respect and reverence for nature are deeply rooted and contribute to a more balanced and conscious life. In Blue Zones, people tend to live in harmony with nature, growing their own food, caring for the land, and enjoying the benefits of a healthy and balanced environment.

The natural environment has a positive impact on longevity.

The natural environment has a positive impact on longevity due to the multiple benefits it provides for physical and mental health. People who live in areas with access to nature, such as parks, forests, mountains, or rural areas, tend to live longer and with a better quality of life. This is due to a combination of key factors that contribute to a healthier and more balanced lifestyle.

One of the main factors is stress reduction. Contact with nature has been shown to be a powerful tool for lowering levels of cortisol, the stress hormone, which in turn reduces the risk of cardiovascular disease, hypertension, and problems related to anxiety and depression.

Nature offers a peaceful and relaxing environment, allowing people to disconnect from the stresses of everyday life and find greater inner peace.

Another important factor is increased physical activity. People who live close to nature tend to be more physically active, as the natural environment encourages activities such as walking, hiking, swimming, and biking. This regular physical activity is essential for maintaining cardiovascular health, improving muscle and bone strength, and reducing the risk of chronic diseases such as type 2 diabetes.

Improved mental health is also a significant benefit of the natural environment. Being surrounded by nature helps reduce anxiety, improves mood, and increases overall well-being. Nature offers a mental respite, allowing the mind to recover from stress and cognitive overload, resulting in greater mental clarity and a better ability to face life's challenges.

Furthermore, contact with the natural environment strengthens the immune system. Plants and trees release beneficial compounds that, when inhaled, help stimulate the immune system, improving the body's ability to fight infections and diseases. This is particularly relevant in preventing chronic diseases and promoting a longer, healthier life.

The culture of prevention in blue zones.

The natural environment has a positive impact on longevity due to the multiple benefits it provides for physical and mental health. People who live in areas with access to nature, such as parks, forests, mountains, or rural areas, tend to live longer and with a better quality of life. This is due to a combination of key factors that contribute to a healthier and more balanced lifestyle.

One of the main factors is stress reduction. Contact with nature has been shown to be a powerful tool for lowering levels of cortisol, the stress hormone, which in turn reduces the risk of cardiovascular disease, hypertension, and problems related to anxiety and depression. Nature offers a peaceful and relaxing environment, allowing people to disconnect from the stresses of everyday life and find greater inner peace.

Another important factor is increased physical activity. People who live close to nature tend to be more physically active, as the natural environment encourages activities such as walking, hiking, swimming, and biking. This regular physical activity is essential for maintaining cardiovascular health, improving muscle and bone strength, and reducing the risk of chronic diseases such as type 2 diabetes.

Improved mental health is also a significant benefit of the natural environment. Being surrounded by nature helps reduce anxiety, improves mood, and increases overall well-being.

Nature offers a mental respite, allowing the mind to recover from stress and cognitive overload, resulting in greater mental clarity and a better ability to face life's challenges.

Furthermore, contact with the natural environment strengthens the immune system. Plants and trees release beneficial compounds that, when inhaled, help stimulate the immune system, improving the body's ability to fight infections and diseases. This is particularly relevant in preventing chronic diseases and promoting a longer, healthier life.

In short, living close to nature encourages an active and healthy lifestyle, which reduces the risk of developing chronic diseases and improves physical and emotional well-being. This more balanced approach to life promotes longevity, allowing people to live longer with a higher quality of life and greater overall well-being.

The culture of prevention in blue zones

The culture of prevention in Blue Zones is one of the key factors contributing to the longevity and exceptional quality of life of the people who live in these regions. Blue Zones, such as Okinawa (Japan), Sardinia (Italy), Ikaria (Greece), Nicoya (Costa Rica), and Loma Linda (United States), are areas of the world where people live longer and healthier lives than the global average.

A central aspect of this longevity is the adoption of preventive habits and practices that not only focus on treating diseases, but also on preventing them from occurring in the first place.

One of the main pillars of the culture of prevention is a healthy and balanced diet, which is naturally integrated into daily life. In the Blue Zones, diets are based primarily on plant-based foods, such as fruits, vegetables, legumes, whole grains, and healthy fats.

These foods are rich in essential nutrients and antioxidants that strengthen the immune system, prevent premature aging, and reduce the risk of chronic diseases such as cardiovascular disease, type 2 diabetes, and cancer. Furthermore, these communities practice moderate portion control, avoiding overindulgence, which also helps prevent overweight and obesity-related diseases.

A focus on regular physical activity is also part of prevention in the Blue Zones. Instead of engaging in strenuous workouts at the gym, people in these regions incorporate movement into their daily lives. Walking long distances, farming, doing housework, and gardening are all activities that keep people consistently active.

This active lifestyle not only strengthens the heart and muscles, but also prevents sedentary lifestyle-related diseases such as cardiovascular problems and osteoporosis. Moderate physical activity also helps maintain flexibility and mobility, which is crucial for maintaining independence in old age.

Another key aspect of prevention in the Blue Zones is stress management. People in these regions have developed daily practices that allow them to naturally reduce stress, such as meditation, daily naps, weekly rest (as in Loma Linda), and connecting with nature.

Chronic stress is a leading cause of cardiovascular disease and immune system disorders, but Blue Zone communities manage to maintain low stress levels through a calm lifestyle, which protects their physical and mental health over the years.

Emotional health also plays an important role in the culture of prevention in the Blue Zones. Close and meaningful interpersonal relationships provide emotional support and a strong sense of community, which contributes to mental well-being and reduces the risk of depression and anxiety.

In Okinawa, for example, the concept of "moai" refers to groups of close friends who support each other throughout life, helping people feel connected and handle life's stress and difficulties in healthier ways.

A sense of purpose is another preventative component that contributes to longevity in these regions. People who have a clear purpose in life, such as taking care of their family, contributing to the community, or continuing to learn and grow, tend to be more emotionally resilient and face life with optimism.

This sense of purpose not only improves mental well-being, but has also been associated with increased longevity, as people stay active, mentally engaged, and motivated to take care of their health.

In addition to these factors, communities in the Blue Zones also have a preventative approach to medical care. Although they do not rely exclusively on modern medicine, people in these regions seek early medical care when necessary and combine traditional medicine with healthy practices that promote prevention.

In Nicoya, for example, people use natural remedies and medicinal plants as part of their health care, helping them prevent disease and maintain ongoing well-being without the need for drastic medical interventions.

The culture of prevention in the Blue Zones is based on a combination of healthy eating, moderate physical activity, stress management, strong social connections, a sense of purpose, and proactive health care. These practices, integrated into daily life, not only prevent disease but also promote a long, full, and high-quality life.

The lessons of the Blue Zones demonstrate that longevity is not just a matter of genetics, but of preventative habits that can be adopted anywhere to improve health and prolong life.

The balance between body and mind

Balance between body and mind is essential for achieving a state of comprehensive well-being, as the two are deeply connected and mutually influence each other. Maintaining this balance is essential for achieving a healthy and fulfilling life, as when the body and mind are in harmony, it helps prevent disease, improves the ability to face challenges, and optimizes performance in all aspects of life.

Achieving this balance involves taking care of both the physical and emotional aspects of our being, adopting practices that promote comprehensive health and long-term well-being.

One of the fundamental pillars of balance between body and mind is regular physical activity, which not only improves physical health but also has a positive impact on mental well-being. Exercise helps release endorphins, known as happiness hormones, which generate a feeling of well-being and reduce stress and anxiety.

Additionally, physical activity improves blood circulation, allowing the brain to receive more oxygen and nutrients, promoting mental clarity and concentration. People who exercise regularly tend to have fewer mental health problems, such as depression and anxiety, as physical movement acts as a natural mood regulator.

Stress management is another crucial component for maintaining balance between body and mind.

Chronic stress affects both the body and mind, weakening the immune system and increasing the risk of diseases such as hypertension, heart disease, and digestive disorders.

Learning to manage stress through techniques such as meditation, deep breathing, and mindfulness helps maintain this balance. Meditation, for example, calms the mind, reduces levels of cortisol (the stress hormone), and improves concentration and focus. Reducing stress also improves physical function, as muscle tension is relieved and an overall state of relaxation is promoted.

Restful sleep is another essential factor in maintaining balance between body and mind. Sleeping well is crucial for the body's recovery and for the mind to process and consolidate the day's information. During sleep, the body regenerates, tissues are repaired, and hormonal balance is restored.

Lack of sleep can negatively affect both physical and mental health, leading to fatigue, irritability, concentration problems, and increased susceptibility to stress. Establishing a proper sleep routine and ensuring you get enough rest each night is essential to maintaining this balance, as the body and mind need time to recover and regenerate.

A balanced diet also plays a key role in maintaining the connection between body and mind. The foods we eat not only affect our physical health but also our mental and emotional well-being. A diet rich in fruits, vegetables, whole grains, legumes, and healthy fats provides the essential nutrients the brain needs to function optimally.

For example, omega-3 fatty acids, found in foods like fish, walnuts, and chia seeds, are essential for brain health and have been shown to have positive effects on mood and cognitive function. Additionally, foods rich in antioxidants and vitamins, such as fresh fruits and vegetables, help reduce inflammation in the body, which in turn improves mental health by lowering the risk of disorders like depression.

Self-awareness is another powerful tool for maintaining balance between body and mind. Being aware of how we feel physically and emotionally allows us to identify when something isn't right and take corrective action before problems worsen.

The practice of Mindfulness is an excellent way to develop this self-awareness. By being present and aware of our emotions and physical sensations, we can respond more effectively to life's demands, rather than reacting impulsively or out of stress. Mindfulness teaches us to listen to the signals from our body and mind, which helps us maintain a constant balance and make adjustments to our self-care routines as needed.

Emotional care. It's also essential for achieving balance between body and mind. Emotional health involves being aware of our emotions, accepting what we feel, and learning to manage them in a healthy way. Ignoring or repressing emotions can lead to both physical and mental imbalance.

Unexpressed or poorly managed emotions can manifest in the body through physical symptoms such as headaches, muscle tension, digestive problems, and fatigue. It's important to learn to recognize negative emotions and find ways to release them, whether through creative expression, dialogue with a trusted friend, or practicing relaxation techniques. By taking care of our emotions, we are also taking care of our bodies, as the two are deeply connected.

The sense of purpose. It's another factor that contributes to the balance between body and mind. People who have a clear purpose in life, whether at work, in relationships, or in their personal activities, tend to experience greater emotional and mental well-being.

Having a reason to get up every morning, whether it's to take care of your family, develop a project, or contribute to the community, provides motivation and energy, which in turn has a positive impact on physical health. A clear purpose helps reduce stress, maintain a positive attitude, and face life's challenges with greater resilience, which promotes balance between body and mind.

Finally, contact with nature is an effective way to restore balance between body and mind. Spending time outdoors, surrounded by trees, mountains, rivers, or the sea, has a restorative effect on both body and mind.

Nature offers a peaceful space where we can disconnect from the stresses of everyday life and reconnect with ourselves. Studies have shown that contact with nature reduces cortisol levels, improves mood, and promotes an overall sense of well-being. People who spend more time in nature tend to experience less stress, fewer mental health problems, and a greater sense of overall well-being.

Balance between body and mind

It is a fundamental aspect of a healthy and fulfilling life. Achieving this balance requires conscious attention to physical, mental, and emotional health, adopting practices that promote the well-being of both body and mind.

Physical activity, stress management, adequate sleep, a balanced diet, self-awareness, emotional care, a sense of purpose, and contact with nature are all factors that contribute to maintaining this balance. When body and mind are in harmony, we not only feel better, but we are also better able to face life's challenges with resilience, energy, and a positive attitude.

The role of a sense of belonging in longevity

A sense of belonging plays a crucial role in longevity and overall well-being, significantly influencing quality of life and the length of life span. This concept refers to the sense of connection and acceptance a person experiences when they are part of a community, social group, or close support network.

Belonging provides us with emotional security, mutual support, and a sense of purpose—all factors that have been linked to increased longevity.

Studies have shown that people who maintain deep interpersonal relationships and a sense of belonging within their communities tend to enjoy better physical and mental health, which contributes to longer and more fulfilling lives.

One of the main effects of a sense of belonging on longevity is stress reduction. People who feel connected to a community and have meaningful relationships tend to experience less stress than those who are isolated or lonely. Chronic stress is one of the factors that most negatively impacts health, as it is linked to problems such as hypertension, heart disease, and immune disorders.

However, by having an emotional support network, people can better cope with life's challenges, as they share their problems and concerns with others, which eases the emotional burden and reduces anxiety. This sense of belonging provides comfort, support, and understanding, allowing people to feel less alone and more capable of handling stressful situations, thereby protecting their health.

In addition to stress reduction, a sense of belonging is linked to the adoption of healthy habits, which contributes to longevity. People who are part of a community tend to adopt healthier lifestyle practices due to the positive influence of their social environment. This can include activities such as exercising in a group, following a balanced diet, or participating in recreational or spiritual activities that promote physical and emotional well-being.

For example, in the Blue Zones, areas where longevity is most common, a sense of community is essential. In Okinawa, Japan, the concept of "moai" brings together groups of friends who support each other throughout life, sharing healthy meals, walks, and moments of reflection. These group activities foster not only physical health but also a sense of belonging and solidarity, which contributes to greater longevity.

The emotional support that comes with a sense of belonging is also key to longevity. People who feel connected to their community are less likely to experience depression and anxiety, two disorders that can seriously affect physical and mental health.

Loneliness and social isolation, on the other hand, are associated with a higher risk of early mortality, as they affect heart health, cognitive function, and the immune system.

Having a group of people with whom to share life's ups and downs creates an emotional buffer that protects against mental and emotional decline.

Close interpersonal relationships help people feel valued and loved, which strengthens their self-esteem and overall well-being.

Another important aspect of belonging is the sense of purpose it brings to people's lives. When someone feels part of a community—whether familial, social, or professional—they usually have a clear purpose that motivates them to continue.

This sense of purpose has been associated with greater longevity, as people who have a clear reason for getting up each morning tend to be more active, resilient, and optimistic.

In Nicoya, Costa Rica, older adults often talk about their "life plan," a concept that gives them direction and a purpose to continue living an active and engaged life, allowing them to stay healthy both physically and mentally. Having a purpose provides intrinsic motivation to take care of oneself and stay engaged in the world, which in turn fosters a longer, more fulfilling life.

A sense of belonging also fosters emotional resilience, a key characteristic for longevity. People who are part of a strong community are better able to bounce back from adversity and trauma.

Resilience is strengthened by connection with others, as the emotional support and practical help provided by the community enable people to overcome difficult situations more easily. This support network acts as a source of strength that helps people cope with grief, illness, or financial hardship, preserving their mental and physical health over time.

By facing challenges with the support of a community, people feel more confident and empowered to move forward, which has a direct impact on their longevity.

Another important factor is that a sense of belonging fosters active and healthy aging. People who feel part of a community tend to be more socially active, which in turn promotes a more dynamic lifestyle.

Participating in social and community activities, such as family gatherings, religious events, clubs, or volunteer groups, not only keeps the body moving, but also stimulates the brain and strengthens interpersonal connections. These social activities help keep the mind sharp and prevent cognitive decline, which is crucial for longevity.

In Blue Zones, older adults are observed to actively participate in the social life of their communities, helping them stay mentally alert and emotionally connected, factors that contribute to their longevity.

Finally, a sense of belonging promotes a positive attitude toward aging. In cultures that value aging and respect their elders, older people tend to feel more valued and appreciated, which has a positive impact on their emotional well-being. When people feel part of a community that recognizes their wisdom and experience, they experience a greater sense of self-worth and life satisfaction.

The positive attitude towards aging

It contributes significantly to better mental health and greater longevity. When people adopt an optimistic view of the aging process, they tend to feel more useful and respected, which has a direct impact on their emotional well-being.

This sense of self-worth not only gives them greater self-esteem but also motivates them to continue taking care of themselves, stay active in their communities, and continue participating in activities that bring them satisfaction and purpose.

Aging is often perceived as a stage in which people lose skills or independence, but when people have a positive attitude toward this phase of life, they tend to see aging as an opportunity to grow, learn, and share experiences.

This attitude fosters emotional resilience, which helps older adults better cope with the challenges and transitions that come with age. Furthermore, feeling valued and respected by their social environment reinforces their sense of belonging and gives them a greater desire to stay involved in activities that benefit both their physical and mental health.

Maintaining a positive attitude toward aging not only improves quality of life, but has also been associated with greater longevity, as those who view this stage favorably are more likely to adopt healthy habits, experience less stress, and maintain an optimistic outlook on the future.

A sense of belonging is crucial for longevity, as it provides emotional support, reduces stress, encourages healthy habits, strengthens resilience, and provides a sense of purpose. People who feel connected to a community tend to live longer and more fully, enjoying better interpersonal relationships, greater life satisfaction, and improved physical and mental health.

Social connection is, therefore, one of the most important pillars for a long and healthy life, and cultivating a sense of belonging is one of the keys to achieving longevity.

Chapter 6.
Proven Strategies to Extend Your Healthy Life

Proven strategies for extending your healthy life are the result of decades of research and observation on how our daily habits influence longevity and quality of life. Living longer depends not only on genetic factors but also on the choices we make throughout our lives, especially regarding diet, physical activity, stress management, and social life.

Consistently incorporating healthy habits can not only extend your life, but also ensure that those additional years are lived with energy, well-being, and fulfillment. Below are science-backed strategies for prolonging your life in a healthy way.

One of the most effective strategies for prolonging life is to follow a balanced diet based on natural foods. Studies have shown that a diet rich in fruits, vegetables, legumes, whole grains, and healthy fats, such as olive oil and nuts, can significantly reduce the risk of chronic diseases such as heart disease, cancer, and type 2 diabetes.

In the Blue Zones, where people live longer than the global average, a predominantly plant-based diet is observed, with limited consumption of meat and processed products. These foods are full of antioxidants, vitamins, minerals, and fiber, which not only nourish the body but also help combat inflammation and oxidative stress, two key factors in aging.

In addition to a healthy diet, moderation in food consumption is another important strategy. Practicing portion control and avoiding overeating can help prevent obesity and obesity-related diseases. In Okinawa, Japan, the "hara hachi bu" principle is practiced, which involves eating until you are 80% full, which helps reduce calorie intake without depriving the body of essential nutrients.

Controlled calorie restriction has been shown to have positive effects on longevity, as it reduces the risk of diseases related to inflammation and slow metabolism, two factors that accelerate aging.

Another crucial strategy for prolonging a healthy life is staying consistently physically active. Regular physical activity is essential for cardiovascular health, muscle strength, and mobility. It's not about performing strenuous exercises, but rather incorporating movement into your daily routine. Walking, biking, gardening, or even doing housework are effective ways to keep your body active without having to go to the gym.

Moderate exercise, performed consistently, improves circulation, strengthens the heart, increases lung capacity, and keeps muscles and bones strong. In Blue Zones, people tend to move naturally throughout the day, whether walking to run errands or working in their gardens, which contributes to their longevity.

Stress management is another key strategy for extending a healthy lifespan. Chronic stress negatively impacts health, increasing the risk of cardiovascular disease, weakening the immune system, and contributing to emotional disorders such as depression and anxiety.

Learning to manage stress through techniques such as meditation, deep breathing, yoga, or mindfulness can significantly reduce these risks. In Ikaria, Greece, for example, daily naps are a common practice that helps reduce stress and improve cardiovascular health. The ability to relax and disconnect from the fast-paced life is essential for prolonging a healthy life.

Adequate sleep is also an essential strategy for a longer, healthier life. Getting seven to nine hours of sleep each night allows the body and mind to regenerate, which is critical for physical and mental health. During sleep, the body repairs tissues, consolidates memory, and regulates hormones that control appetite, stress, and metabolism.

Lack of adequate sleep can increase the risk of chronic diseases such as diabetes and hypertension, as well as negatively affect mood and cognitive function. Establishing a healthy sleep routine, avoiding the use of electronic devices before bed, and creating an environment conducive to rest are essential for improving the quality and quantity of life.

Another proven strategy for extending life is maintaining meaningful interpersonal relationships. Emotional and social support is crucial for mental and emotional well-being, and research shows that people with strong social relationships tend to live longer. In Blue Zones, a sense of community and interpersonal connections are key to longevity.

In Okinawa, the concept of "moai" brings together groups of friends who support each other throughout life, providing a consistent support network that reduces stress and fosters emotional well-being. People who feel connected and supported by their community experience less loneliness and depression, which contributes to better mental and physical health over the years.

A sense of purpose is also essential for extending life in a healthy way. People who have a clear purpose in life, such as caring for family, contributing to the community, or continuing to learn and develop, tend to live longer and in better health.

Purpose provides a reason to get up every morning and stay active, both physically and mentally. In Nicoya, Costa Rica, older adults talk about their "life plan," which gives them direction and motivation to continue living active and fulfilling lives. Having a purpose not only improves emotional well-being but also reduces the risk of stress-related illnesses and inactivity.

Contact with nature is another important strategy for prolonging a healthy life. Spending time outdoors, surrounded by nature, reduces stress, improves mood, and promotes a greater sense of overall well-being. Nature offers a tranquil space where people can relax, disconnect from the stresses of daily life, and recharge.

Furthermore, exposure to sunlight is essential for the production of vitamin D, which is crucial for bone health and the immune system. Spending time in nature also encourages physical activity, such as walking or hiking, which contributes to a longer, healthier life.

Finally, a positive attitude toward life is a fundamental strategy for extending longevity. People who maintain an optimistic outlook on aging and life in general tend to be more resilient and better able to cope with challenges. A positive attitude reduces stress, improves emotional well-being, and fosters healthy habits.

Optimistic people tend to take better care of themselves, eat well, exercise, and maintain positive interpersonal relationships, all of which contribute to a longer, better-quality life.

In conclusion, proven strategies for extending a healthy life include a combination of healthy habits that encompass nutrition, physical activity, stress management, adequate sleep, interpersonal relationships, a sense of purpose, contact with nature, and a positive attitude.

These practices, adopted consistently over time, not only prolong life but also ensure that those additional years are lived with vitality, energy, and overall well-being. The lessons learned from long-lived individuals in the Blue Zones show us that living longer isn't just a matter of luck, but of adopting daily habits that promote a life rich in health and satisfaction.

The importance of intermittent fasting and calorie restriction

Intermittent fasting and calorie restriction are two practices that have gained popularity in recent years due to their positive impact on health and longevity.

Although they are related concepts, they have key differences, but both are based on principles that promote reducing food intake over certain periods of time or generally limiting calories consumed.

Scientific studies have shown that both intermittent fasting and calorie restriction can offer a wide range of health benefits, from weight loss to improved metabolism, cell regeneration, and the prevention of chronic diseases. These practices not only promote a healthier life but have also been linked to increased longevity.

Intermittent fasting is an eating pattern that alternates between periods of fasting and eating. Instead of focusing on what to eat, it focuses more on when to eat.

There are different forms of intermittent fasting, the most common being the 16:8 method, in which you fast for 16 hours and concentrate your food intake in an 8-hour window, and the 5:2 method, where you eat normally for 5 days and drastically reduce your calorie intake for 2 days a week.

Intermittent fasting allows the body time to rest from the digestion process and use stored energy, which activates a series of biological processes that benefit health.

One of the main benefits of intermittent fasting is its ability to improve insulin sensitivity. When we eat frequently, the body is constantly processing glucose, which can lead to insulin resistance, a key risk factor for type 2 diabetes.

However, during periods of fasting, insulin levels decrease and the body begins to use fat stores as an energy source, which improves insulin sensitivity and helps regulate blood glucose levels. This not only prevents diabetes but also reduces the risk of heart disease, obesity, and other metabolic disorders.

Intermittent fasting also stimulates the process of autophagy, an essential cellular mechanism for the regeneration and maintenance of healthy cells.

During periods of fasting, the body initiates autophagy, a process in which cells degrade and recycle their damaged or dysfunctional components. This process is crucial for removing damaged proteins and organelles that can accumulate over time and contribute to aging and the development of diseases like cancer and Alzheimer's. By activating autophagy, intermittent fasting helps keep cells healthy and promotes longevity.

Improvements in brain function.

Furthermore, intermittent fasting is associated with improvements in brain function. Studies have shown that intermittent fasting can increase the production of a protein called brain-derived neurotrophic factor (BDNF), which is essential for the growth and survival of neurons.

This increase in BDNF improves cognitive function, protects the brain against neurodegenerative diseases, and promotes brain plasticity, which is crucial for maintaining good mental health over the years. Intermittent fasting has also been observed to reduce inflammation in the brain, which contributes to the prevention of disorders such as depression and Alzheimer's.

On the other hand, calorie restriction is the practice of reducing total calorie intake without becoming malnourished. Unlike intermittent fasting, which is based on cycles of eating and fasting, calorie restriction involves consistently consuming fewer calories while ensuring the body receives the necessary nutrients. Numerous animal and human studies have shown that calorie restriction can extend lifespan and reduce the risk of chronic diseases, such as heart disease, cancer, and diabetes.

One of the most notable effects of calorie restriction is its ability to reduce oxidative stress in the body. Oxidative stress is a process in which free radicals damage cells and tissues, contributing to aging and the development of chronic diseases.

Calorie restriction reduces the production of free radicals, helping to protect cells from damage and keep them functioning properly for longer. This is critical for preventing premature aging and improving longevity.

Another important benefit of calorie restriction is its ability to improve cardiovascular health. Consuming fewer calories reduces blood pressure, improves cholesterol levels, and decreases the risk of developing arteriosclerosis, a condition in which the arteries harden due to fatty buildup. Maintaining a healthy cardiovascular system reduces the risk of heart attacks, strokes, and other problems associated with aging.

Reducing chronic inflammation is another key benefit of both intermittent fasting and calorie restriction. Chronic inflammation is linked to a wide variety of diseases, including heart disease, cancer, and neurodegenerative disorders. By reducing calorie intake and providing digestive rest periods, the body can reduce inflammation levels, promoting better overall health and reducing the risk of developing these diseases over time.

Furthermore, calorie restriction has also been shown to have positive effects on increasing longevity. In animal studies, those who consumed fewer calories lived longer and had fewer age-related diseases.

Although human results are still being investigated, early evidence suggests that calorie restriction could have similar effects in humans, delaying cellular aging and improving overall health.

On a mental level, calorie restriction can also have significant benefits. Reducing calorie intake has been observed to improve mood and reduce symptoms of anxiety and depression.

This could be related to the fact that consuming fewer calories stimulates the production of hormones and neurotransmitters that improve mental health, such as serotonin and endorphins.

So, both intermittent fasting and calorie restriction are science-backed strategies that can significantly improve health and promote longevity.

By reducing caloric intake and allowing the body to rest from digestion, these practices help improve metabolism, promote autophagy, reduce oxidative stress and inflammation, and prevent a host of chronic diseases.

Furthermore, their benefits for brain, cardiovascular, and emotional health contribute to improving quality of life over time. Incorporating these strategies in a balanced and sustainable way into daily life can be a powerful tool for living longer and healthier lives.

Controlling chronic diseases through lifestyle habits.

This control is a fundamental strategy for improving health and quality of life, as well as preventing serious complications. Chronic diseases, such as type 2 diabetes, hypertension, heart disease, obesity, and some types of cancer, are the leading causes of death worldwide.

Although many factors, such as genetics and age, can influence the development of these diseases, healthy lifestyle habits have been shown to play a crucial role in their prevention, management, and control. Adopting a lifestyle based on a balanced diet, regular exercise, stress reduction, adequate rest, and avoiding harmful habits can make a significant difference in the management and progression of chronic diseases.

One of the most important pillars for managing chronic diseases is a healthy diet. Diet has a direct impact on the prevention and management of diseases such as diabetes, cardiovascular disease, and hypertension. Consuming a diet rich in fruits, vegetables, whole grains, legumes, and healthy fats, such as those found in olive oil and nuts, provides essential nutrients for optimal body function.

These foods are rich in antioxidants, fiber, vitamins, and minerals, which help reduce inflammation and prevent cell damage, both key factors in the development of chronic diseases.

In particular, a diet low in sugars and refined carbohydrates is critical for managing type 2 diabetes. Excess sugar in the diet can cause blood glucose spikes and increase insulin resistance, which worsens diabetes and contributes to other health complications. Choosing complex carbohydrates, such as those found in whole grains, and limiting processed foods and sugary drinks helps keep blood sugar levels stable.

Additionally, consuming fiber-rich foods, such as fruits, vegetables, and legumes, improves digestion and slows glucose absorption, which is beneficial for managing diabetes.

When it comes to heart disease and hypertension, reducing sodium and saturated fat intake is essential. Excess salt in the diet is linked to increased blood pressure, which can lead to hypertension, a key risk factor for heart disease and stroke.

Incorporating potassium-rich foods, such as bananas, spinach, and potatoes, can counteract the effects of sodium and help maintain healthy blood pressure levels.

Additionally, choosing healthy fats like those found in olive oil, avocado, and nuts instead of saturated and trans fats (found in processed and fried foods) improves cardiovascular health by reducing LDL cholesterol ("bad" cholesterol) levels and increasing HDL cholesterol ("good" cholesterol) levels.

Regular physical exercise is another crucial component for managing chronic diseases.

Physical activity improves cardiovascular health, reduces the risk of obesity, improves insulin sensitivity, and lowers blood pressure.

Moderate aerobic exercise, such as walking, swimming, or cycling, has been shown to be especially beneficial for managing conditions such as diabetes, hypertension, and heart disease. Regular movement helps burn calories, which contributes to losing or maintaining a healthy weight, reduces visceral fat (which is linked to the risk of chronic disease), and improves blood circulation.

Additionally, exercise helps strengthen the heart and improve its ability to pump blood more efficiently, which is crucial for maintaining proper blood pressure.

For people with diabetes, exercise is particularly important because it helps improve the body's ability to use glucose as an energy source, which lowers blood sugar levels and improves insulin sensitivity. Exercise also contributes to weight loss, which can be especially beneficial for people with type 2 diabetes, as excess weight is one of the main risk factors for the disease.

Stress management is another crucial factor in managing chronic diseases. Chronic stress can negatively affect both physical and mental health and is linked to an increased risk of developing cardiovascular disease, diabetes, and metabolic disorders.

Stress triggers the release of hormones like cortisol and adrenaline, which increase blood pressure and blood glucose levels, worsening conditions like hypertension and diabetes. Learning to manage stress through techniques like meditation, yoga, deep breathing, and mindfulness can help reduce these negative effects.

Meditation, for example, not only reduces cortisol levels, but also improves mental clarity and promotes an overall state of relaxation, which benefits both the mind and body.

Adequate rest is also critical for managing chronic diseases. Sleep allows the body to regenerate and repair, which is crucial for hormonal regulation and managing conditions such as diabetes, hypertension, and cardiovascular disease. Lack of sleep is linked to an increased risk of obesity, as it disrupts the hormones that control hunger and appetite, leading to overeating and weight gain.

Additionally, lack of sleep affects insulin sensitivity, worsening type 2 diabetes. Getting between 7 and 9 hours of sleep per night is essential for maintaining proper hormonal balance and improving physical and mental health.

Another key habit for managing chronic diseases is abstaining from harmful habits, such as smoking and excessive alcohol consumption. Tobacco is one of the main risk factors for developing heart disease, cancer, and chronic respiratory diseases, as it damages arteries, raises blood pressure, and increases the risk of blood clots.

Quitting tobacco not only improves cardiovascular health, but also reduces the risk of lung cancer and improves lung capacity, which is crucial for people with respiratory diseases. As for alcohol, excessive consumption can raise blood pressure, increase triglyceride levels, and contribute to the accumulation of abdominal fat, which worsens chronic diseases.

Drinking in moderation, or avoiding it altogether, can have positive effects on long-term health.

Finally, social support is another important factor in managing chronic illnesses. People who have a supportive network, whether family, friends, or support groups, tend to have better outcomes in managing their illnesses.

Emotional and social support helps reduce stress, improves adherence to treatment, and promotes healthier lifestyle habits. Furthermore, people with social support tend to be more physically active and better follow medical recommendations, which improves the management of chronic conditions.

In short, chronic disease control through lifestyle choices is possible by adopting a healthy diet, exercising regularly, managing stress, getting adequate rest, and avoiding harmful habits. These lifestyle changes not only improve quality of life but also reduce the risk of serious complications and promote greater longevity.

Although chronic diseases can be difficult to manage, adopting healthy habits is an effective strategy for improving health and living a full and active life.

Social Connection: How Mutual Support Strengthens Health.

Social connection and mutual support are fundamental factors that influence people's health and well-being. Numerous studies have shown that strong interpersonal relationships and a sense of belonging to a community not only improve mental and emotional health but also have a direct impact on physical health.

Mutual support, which includes both giving and receiving emotional, material, or practical support, strengthens resilience in the face of difficulties, improves the ability to cope with stress, and, in the long run, contributes to a healthier and longer life.

In an increasingly interconnected, yet individualized, world, maintaining and strengthening social connections has become crucial to promoting a full and balanced life.

One of the clearest benefits of social connection is its ability to reduce stress. People who have a support network, whether through friends, family, or colleagues, tend to cope better with life's challenges.

Sharing problems and concerns with others not only eases the emotional burden but also offers new perspectives and solutions, reducing anxiety and stress levels. Chronic stress is linked to a host of health problems, including heart disease, hypertension, and immune disorders. However, when people receive emotional support, their bodies respond better to stress, releasing less cortisol, the stress hormone, and maintaining a more balanced state both physically and mentally.

Mutual support also has a significant impact on mental health. Maintaining close, meaningful relationships provides a sense of belonging and emotional security, which reduces the risk of developing mental disorders such as depression and anxiety.

Loneliness and social isolation, on the other hand, are associated with an increased risk of depression, anxiety, and other mental health problems. When people feel connected to others and part of a community, they are more likely to experience positive emotions, such as happiness, life satisfaction, and a greater sense of purpose.

This emotional well-being, in turn, has beneficial effects on physical health, as it reduces inflammation, improves immune function, and protects the cardiovascular system.

Another crucial aspect of social connection is its ability to foster healthy lifestyle habits. People who are part of strong social networks tend to adopt healthier behaviors, such as exercising regularly, eating a balanced diet, and avoiding harmful habits like smoking or excessive alcohol consumption.

Mutual support not only motivates people to take care of themselves, but also facilitates access to resources and knowledge that promote healthier lives. For example, in communities where a sense of belonging is strong, such as in Blue Zones—regions of the world where people live longer and with a better quality of life—friends and family play an active role in encouraging one another to maintain healthy lifestyles, which contributes to longevity.

Furthermore, social support is linked to improved cardiovascular health. Studies have shown that people with strong social connections are less likely to develop heart disease or suffer a stroke.

This is due, in part, to reduced stress and lower blood pressure, but also to the positive effects of social support on the adoption of healthy behaviors. People who feel supported by their social environment tend to be more motivated to take care of their health and follow medical recommendations, which includes controlling their blood pressure, reducing cholesterol, and maintaining a healthy weight—key factors in preventing cardiovascular disease.

Mutual support also strengthens emotional resilience and resilience in the face of life's challenges. People with a strong support network are better able to cope with difficult situations, such as grief, job loss, or health problems.

The emotional support provided by social connection acts as a "cushion" that cushions the emotional impact of adversity, allowing people to recover more quickly and with fewer aftereffects. This resilience is crucial not only for mental health but also for physical health, as it reduces the likelihood that chronic stress will affect the immune system and other vital body systems.

The sense of belonging that arises from social connection also provides purpose and direction in life. Feeling part of a community or having meaningful relationships gives people a reason to get up every day, which is directly related to greater longevity.

In Okinawa, Japan, for example, residents practice "ikigai," which translates as "the reason for living," "the purpose." This sense of purpose is shared and strengthened through social connections and helps people stay physically and mentally active, which contributes to their longevity.

Personal purpose not only improves emotional well-being, but also encourages healthy habits and reduces the risk of aging-related diseases.

Another way in which social connection benefits health is by strengthening the immune system. Studies suggest that people with a strong social network have a better immune response and are more resistant to infections.

This is because emotional support reduces chronic stress, which weakens the immune system, and fosters a positive state of mind, which is linked to increased production of immune cells. People who feel emotionally supported are less likely to get sick, and when they do, they tend to recover faster than those who experience loneliness or social isolation.

Furthermore, social connection is especially important for healthy aging. As people age, maintaining close and meaningful interpersonal relationships is critical to preventing loneliness and isolation, which are risk factors for cognitive decline and neurodegenerative diseases.

Older adults who remain involved in their communities and maintain active relationships with family and friends tend to be more mentally agile and have a lower risk of developing diseases such as Alzheimer's.

Social activities also stimulate the mind, promote intellectual curiosity, and provide a sense of purpose—all key factors for healthy aging.

Finally, social connection and mutual support foster a collaborative approach to well-being. By connecting with people who share similar values and goals, people feel more motivated to participate in activities that improve their well-being, such as playing group sports, attending meditation classes, or participating in community activities.

These shared experiences not only strengthen social ties but also create a positive environment where people feel supported in their efforts to maintain good health. Collaboration and mutual support make it easier to adopt and maintain healthy lifestyle habits, which contributes to a longer and more well-being life.

Social connection and mutual support are essential for promoting good physical, mental, and emotional health. Strong interpersonal relationships provide emotional support, reduce stress, encourage healthy lifestyle habits, and strengthen resilience in the face of life's challenges.

These connections not only improve quality of life but are also linked to greater longevity and better overall health.

In a world where social isolation and loneliness are increasingly common, it's more important than ever to cultivate and maintain meaningful relationships that allow us to thrive and live life to the fullest.

The power of purpose, ikigai in long-lived cultures.

The power of purpose is a key factor that directly influences people's longevity and quality of life, and this concept is notably reflected in ikigai, a Japanese term meaning "the reason for being" or "the reason for getting up every morning."

Ikigai is a fundamental pillar of long-lived cultures, especially in Okinawa, Japan, one of the regions known as the Blue Zones, where people live longer and healthier than the global average.

The concept of ikigai not only encompasses work or professional goals but also includes any activity or connection that brings meaning and satisfaction to everyday life, from personal relationships to healthcare.

This approach to life, deeply rooted in long-lived communities, highlights how having a clear purpose can improve physical, mental, and emotional well-being, and how that purpose can significantly extend life.

Ikigai is a central concept in longevity because it provides people with an intrinsic motivation to keep going, regardless of age. In longevity cultures like Okinawa's, ikigai refers to the idea that each individual has a special mission or reason for living, whether it's caring for family, gardening, participating in community activities, or continuing to learn and explore new interests.

This sense of purpose gives them a reason to stay active and engaged in life, which, in turn, promotes healthy habits and a positive attitude toward aging. People with strong ikigai tend to enjoy greater life satisfaction, less stress, and greater emotional resilience, all of which contribute to a longer, more fulfilling life.

One of the most powerful aspects of ikigai is its impact on mental health. People who have a clear sense of purpose tend to experience less anxiety and depression, as they feel connected to something larger than themselves.

This purpose gives them a framework for interpreting life events, including difficulties, from a positive and meaningful perspective. Rather than getting caught up in negative thoughts or worries about aging, people with a strong ikigai tend to view life as a continuous opportunity to contribute and grow.

This sense of meaning also reduces the perception of stress, which improves mental health and protects the brain from the negative effects of chronic stress, such as mental fatigue, anxiety, and depression.

Ikigai also has a direct impact on physical health. Purpose in life motivates people to take better care of their bodies and stay active longer. In Okinawa, for example, many elderly people continue to work in their gardens, walk long distances, and engage in light physical activity every day, not because it's an obligation, but because they see it as part of their life purpose.

This natural approach to physical activity not only strengthens the body but also improves cardiovascular health, reduces the risk of chronic diseases such as diabetes and hypertension, and maintains mobility throughout the years. Deeply connected to their ikigai, Okinawans view old age not as a period of decline, but as an opportunity to continue contributing and living actively.

Another important aspect of ikigai is that it fosters meaningful interpersonal relationships. Part of the purpose of many people in long-lived cultures is related to caring for others, whether within the family, circle of friends, or the wider community. Ikigai encourages people to nurture their social relationships, which, in turn, provides them with emotional support and a greater sense of belonging.

In Okinawa, the concept of "moai" is a good example of how ikigai is connected to interpersonal relationships.

Moai are groups of close friends who support each other throughout their lives, and this support network provides a sense of purpose and emotional security, helping to reduce stress and improve mental and physical health. People who feel connected and valued within a community are less likely to experience loneliness, a factor that has been linked to an increased risk of premature mortality and mental health problems.

The power of purpose. It also extends to people's ability to face and overcome adversity. Having a strong ikigai provides an internal source of motivation that helps people cope with difficult times and find meaning in even the most challenging situations.

In long-lived cultures, older adults with a clear purpose in life tend to display greater emotional resilience and a better ability to adapt to the inevitable changes that aging brings. This resilience not only allows them to maintain a positive attitude in the face of difficulties, but also has a direct impact on their physical health, as chronic stress and a lack of purpose are linked to health decline.

Ikigai is also linked to a positive attitude toward aging. In many cultures, aging is perceived as a time of decline and loss, which can lead to a decrease in emotional well-being and motivation to continue taking care of one's health. However, in long-lived cultures that value ikigai, aging is seen as an opportunity to continue contributing to community and family, which promotes a sense of worth and an optimistic attitude toward advanced years.

This positive mindset not only improves quality of life, but has also been linked to increased longevity, as people who view aging favorably tend to take better care of themselves, stay active, and experience less stress.

The power of ikigai also manifests itself in people's ability to continue learning and developing throughout their lives. Having a clear purpose motivates people to stay mentally active and continue challenging themselves, which is critical for maintaining cognitive acuity and preventing age-related mental decline.

People with strong ikigai tend to seek out new experiences, continue learning, and engage in mentally stimulating activities, which helps them stay mentally sharp and reduce their risk of neurodegenerative diseases, such as Alzheimer's.

This constant commitment to personal growth and intellectual curiosity is a key factor in maintaining cognitive health throughout life. By having a clear purpose that motivates them, these people remain mentally active, challenging themselves with new tasks, acquiring skills, and exploring different interests.

This cognitive stimulation not only keeps the brain functioning optimally, but also contributes to the creation of new neural connections, a protective factor against cognitive decline and age-related diseases such as Alzheimer's.

By providing a sense of purpose and direction, ikigai fosters a mindset of continuous growth that supports both longevity and mental well-being.

This focus on continuous learning and personal growth is one of the key factors contributing to longevity in the Blue Zones.

The power of purpose, exemplified by the concept of ikigai in long-lived cultures, is an essential element for a long and healthy life. Having a clear purpose provides motivation, emotional resilience, and a reason to stay active and engaged in life, which improves both physical and mental health.

Ikigai not only fosters healthy habits and meaningful relationships, but also offers an internal source of satisfaction and well-being that helps people age gracefully, with optimism, and a sense of fulfillment.

In long-lived cultures, ikigai is a powerful force that not only extends life, but ensures that those additional years are lived with purpose, meaning, and a deep connection to community and the world.

Chapter 7.
How Blue Zones Inspire a Healthy Approach to Longevity

Blue Zones are regions of the world where people live significantly longer and healthier lives than elsewhere. These areas include Okinawa (Japan), Sardinia (Italy), Ikaria (Greece), the Nicoya Peninsula (Costa Rica), and Loma Linda (California, USA).

In these communities, life expectancy is higher, and rates of chronic diseases such as diabetes, heart disease, and cancer are remarkably low. Residents of Blue Zones not only live longer, but also experience a better quality of life in their later years, remaining active, mentally agile, and socially connected.

The lifestyle approach practiced in these regions has inspired health and wellness experts to identify habits and lifestyles that promote healthy and sustainable longevity.

One of the most inspiring aspects of the Blue Zones is their focus on plant-based eating. Diets in these regions are characterized by a high consumption of fresh, whole, and unprocessed foods, especially fruits, vegetables, legumes, whole grains, and healthy fats like olive oil and nuts.

Meat, processed foods, and refined sugar are consumed in minimal or moderate amounts. In Ikaria, Greece, for example, the Mediterranean diet is based on olive oil, fresh vegetables, legumes, and the occasional fish. This type of diet is packed with antioxidants, vitamins, minerals, and fiber, which not only promote cardiovascular health but also reduce the risk of chronic diseases and strengthen the immune system.

The Blue Zones diet inspires a balanced approach to nutrition that prioritizes natural, plant-based foods, resulting in greater longevity.

Another key factor inspiring a healthy approach to longevity in the Blue Zones is consistent but moderate physical activity. Unlike Western approaches that focus on intense, structured exercise, people in these regions naturally integrate movement into their daily lives.

Walking, gardening, caring for the family, and doing household chores are common activities that keep people physically active throughout their lives. In Sardinia, Italy, shepherds walk long distances in mountainous terrain every day, which allows them to maintain excellent cardiovascular and muscular health.

This approach to physical activity is accessible to people of all ages, ensuring that Blue Zone residents remain active, mobile, and functional even in old age. The key isn't extreme exercise, but rather consistent daily movement.

Stress management is also a key component of longevity in Blue Zones. People living in these regions have developed daily practices that help them reduce stress and stay emotionally balanced.

In Icaria, daily siestas are part of the routine, allowing people to rest and disconnect from the pressures of everyday life.

Effective stress management helps prevent chronic stress-related health problems, such as heart disease and hypertension, and promotes greater emotional well-being. The lessons of the Blue Zones in this regard inspire the adoption of stress-reducing self-care practices, such as meditation, deep breathing, or simply taking regular breaks to relax.

The sense of community and social support is another inspiring aspect of longevity in Blue Zones. People in these regions have strong social connections, live surrounded by family and friends, and are actively involved in their communities. This sense of belonging and mutual support provides them with an emotional safety net that helps them better manage life's challenges, such as illness or loss.

Deep interpersonal relationships reduce stress, improve mental and emotional health, and foster a greater sense of purpose and satisfaction.

Social support is essential for longevity, as people who feel connected and supported are less likely to suffer from depression, loneliness, and anxiety, which has a direct impact on their physical health.

Furthermore, people in Blue Zones have a strong sense of purpose, which motivates them to remain active and engaged in life throughout the years. This purpose, known as "ikigai" in Okinawa, Japan, or "life plan" in Nicoya, Costa

Rica, gives them a reason to get up every day and continue contributing to their families and communities.

Having a clear purpose has been linked to greater longevity, as it provides motivation and energy to continue taking care of one's physical and mental health. People with a sense of purpose tend to face aging with a positive attitude, which helps them stay active and mentally agile.

Adequate rest is also a crucial element in the Blue Zones. Getting enough sleep allows the body to regenerate, the immune system to strengthen, and the brain to process the day's information. Quality rest is essential for longevity, as lack of sleep is associated with a higher incidence of chronic diseases such as diabetes, hypertension, and heart disease.

In the Blue Zones, rest not only refers to nighttime sleep, but also to regular breaks during the day to relax and unwind, such as siestas in Ikaria. This approach balances activity with rest, promoting overall well-being.

Finally, balance and moderation are key principles in the Blue Zones that inspire a healthy approach to longevity. People in these regions practice moderation in all areas of their lives, from nutrition to work and rest.

Practicing moderation not only helps maintain a healthy weight, but also reduces the risk of chronic diseases and promotes a longer life.

The Blue Zones inspire a holistic and balanced approach to longevity, based on simple yet powerful habits that promote a long, healthy, and fulfilling life. A plant-based diet, consistent physical activity, stress management, a sense of community, a sense of purpose, adequate rest, and moderation are the key principles that guide these longevity cultures.

These lessons offer a clear model of how small lifestyle changes can have a profound impact on health and quality of life as we age. By adopting these habits, it's possible not only to live longer, but also to enjoy those years with vitality and well-being.

The holistic approach to health in the blue zones

The holistic approach to health in Blue Zones is one of the fundamental pillars that contribute to the longevity and overall well-being of people living in these regions. Blue Zones, such as Okinawa in Japan, Sardinia in Italy, Ikaria in Greece, the Nicoya Peninsula in Costa Rica, and Loma Linda in the United States, are areas where people not only live longer but also enjoy a better quality of life throughout their years.

Unlike fragmented approaches that tend to separate the physical, mental, and emotional aspects of health, the holistic Blue Zones approach treats the individual as a whole, integrating diverse aspects of daily life to maintain balance and harmony in body, mind, and spirit.

This comprehensive approach is based on a combination of healthy habits, strong social connections, a balanced diet, consistent physical activity, and effective stress management, all framed within a deep sense of purpose and community well-being.

One of the most important elements of the holistic approach in the Blue Zones is a balanced diet, which focuses on natural foods, primarily of plant origin, and avoids ultra-processed products.

People in these regions consume primarily fruits, vegetables, legumes, whole grains, and healthy fats, such as olive oil and nuts.

In Okinawa, for example, the diet includes abundant amounts of green leafy vegetables, sweet potatoes, and tofu, while in Ikaria and Sardinia, the Mediterranean diet is rich in legumes, olive oil, fish, and a moderate amount of meat.

This dietary approach not only ensures adequate intake of essential nutrients, but also promotes cardiovascular health and reduces the risk of chronic diseases such as diabetes and cancer.

Furthermore, practicing moderation in eating, such as the "hara hachi bu" in Okinawa, which involves eating only until you are 80% full, prevents excess calories and promotes a healthy weight throughout life.

In addition to nutrition, moderate but consistent physical activity is another pillar of the holistic approach to health in the Blue Zones. In these regions, exercise is not perceived as a mandatory or intense task, but is naturally integrated into daily life.

Walking long distances, gardening, doing household chores, or actively moving from one place to another are examples of how Blue Zone residents keep their bodies moving regularly.

In Sardinia, shepherds walk for miles through mountainous terrain as part of their daily routine, which helps maintain good cardiovascular and muscular health without the need for strenuous exercise.

This constant but non-exhausting physical activity is key to keeping the body agile and strong throughout life, reducing the risk of sedentary lifestyle-related diseases such as obesity and hypertension.

Stress management is also an essential aspect of the holistic approach to health in the Blue Zones. People in these regions have developed effective strategies to reduce stress and promote emotional calm. In Ikaria, Greece, taking naps is a daily practice that allows them to unwind and relax, helping to reduce levels of cortisol, the stress hormone.

In Loma Linda, Seventh-day Adventists practice weekly rest by devoting a full day to spirituality, rest, and reflection, as we have mentioned before.

This regular disconnection from daily demands helps protect the body from the damaging effects of chronic stress, such as inflammation, hypertension, and mental health issues. The holistic approach in the Blue Zones teaches that managing stress is just as important as caring for the physical body, and so people continually seek ways to balance their mind and spirit with relaxation techniques and practices that promote inner peace.

A key component of the holistic approach in Blue Zones is a sense of community and strong social connections. Deep and meaningful interpersonal relationships are fundamental to the well-being of people living in these regions. Social life in Blue Zones is marked by a strong sense of belonging and mutual support.

In Okinawa, for example, people form groups of friends known as "moai," who support each other throughout life.

These social connections provide emotional support, which reduces the risk of illnesses related to isolation and loneliness, such as depression and anxiety. Interpersonal relationships in these communities also foster a sense of security and peace of mind, which contributes to greater emotional stability.

In Sardinia, older adults are respected and valued by their families and communities, which strengthens their self-esteem and provides them with a continued purpose in life.

A sense of purpose is intrinsically linked to longevity, as it provides people with a constant source of motivation and personal satisfaction. Having a purpose in life not only improves emotional well-being but also encourages healthy habits and reduces stress. People with a clear purpose tend to stay more active and engaged, which contributes to a longer, better-quality life.

Adequate rest is another fundamental element of the holistic approach to health in the Blue Zones. Getting enough sleep each night allows the body to regenerate and repair, which is crucial for maintaining a strong immune system and a healthy brain. Lack of sleep is linked to a number of health problems, including obesity, diabetes, and heart disease.

In the Blue Zones, rest not only refers to nighttime sleep, but also the ability to take breaks during the day to relax and recharge. A balance between activity and rest is essential for maintaining physical and mental health over the years.

The holistic approach to health in the Blue Zones also extends to spirituality and connection with nature. At Loma Linda, Seventh-day Adventists not only promote a healthy diet and rest, but also practice spirituality as a way to connect with something greater than themselves. This spiritual connection offers a sense of peace, purpose, and belonging that strengthens emotional and mental well-being.

Similarly, contact with nature in regions like Icaria and Nicoya has a restorative effect. Spending time outdoors, surrounded by mountains, oceans, or gardens, helps reduce stress, improve mood, and strengthen the body.

Thus, the holistic approach to health in the Blue Zones is based on the integration of various aspects of daily life to achieve a complete balance between body, mind, and spirit. The combination of a balanced diet, moderate physical activity, stress management, meaningful social relationships, a clear sense of purpose, and adequate rest, along with a spiritual and natural connection, creates a powerful formula for a long and healthy life.

This holistic approach to health not only improves quality of life but also offers a model for how small lifestyle changes can have a profound impact on longevity and overall well-being. The lessons of the Blue Zones show us that a full and long life is possible when we treat the individual as a whole, caring for all aspects of their being.

The influence of spirituality on longevity.

The influence of spirituality on longevity is a deeply studied topic that highlights the relationship between spiritual practices, emotional and physical well-being, and life extension. Although spirituality can be expressed in diverse ways across cultures and beliefs, its impact on health is significant.

Spirituality not only offers emotional and mental comfort but also promotes a balanced approach to life, including stress reduction, resilience building, strong social bonds, and, in many cases, healthy lifestyle habits.

These dimensions, when integrated, contribute to greater longevity, offering a more balanced and meaningful life.

One of the most influential factors of spirituality in longevity is its ability to reduce stress. People who practice some form of spirituality, whether through prayer, meditation, yoga, or participation in religious rituals, tend to experience lower levels of anxiety and stress.

Spirituality provides a transcendental perspective that helps people see everyday problems from a broader perspective. By trusting in a higher power or a greater purpose, people develop a greater capacity to accept difficulties with serenity and less anxiety.

This translates into lower levels of cortisol, the stress hormone, which, in excess, is associated with chronic health problems such as heart disease, hypertension, and immune disorders. By reducing chronic stress, spirituality protects physical and mental health, promoting a longer life.

Emotional resilience

Spirituality is also deeply linked to emotional resilience, which is crucial for longevity. People who practice spirituality tend to find meaning and purpose even in difficult situations. In many spiritual traditions, suffering is viewed as an opportunity for growth or as part of a divine plan, allowing believers to face difficulties with greater strength.

This ability to find meaning in difficult times helps them recover more quickly from emotional shocks and maintain a positive attitude, which has a direct impact on their health. Emotional resilience protects against the negative effects of prolonged stress, resulting in improved immune function, greater emotional stability, and, consequently, greater longevity.

Another important factor in the influence of spirituality on longevity is that many spiritual traditions promote healthy lifestyle habits. Religious and spiritual practices often encourage their followers to adopt healthier lifestyles, including balanced diets, abstaining from alcohol and tobacco, and practicing adequate rest.

A clear example is the Seventh-day Adventist community in Loma Linda, California, one of the Blue Zones, where people live significantly longer than average. This community follows a predominantly vegetarian diet, avoids the use of harmful substances, and observes a full day of rest each week, which reduces stress and promotes spiritual reflection.

These practices not only improve physical health by preventing chronic diseases, but also provide emotional and mental balance that contributes to longevity.

Spirituality is also closely linked to developing strong social connections, a key factor in longevity. People who participate in spiritual or religious communities tend to have stronger emotional support networks, which provides them with a sense of belonging and emotional security.

Research shows that people with deep and meaningful social connections are less likely to suffer from depression, anxiety, and loneliness, factors linked to poor physical and mental health. Spiritual communities often foster mutual care, which strengthens social bonds and contributes to emotional well-being.

These interpersonal connections are essential for longevity, as emotional and social support reduces stress levels, improves immune function, and helps people better cope with life's challenges.

A sense of purpose is another dimension of spirituality that has a notable influence on longevity. Many spiritual traditions teach that life has a purpose beyond material or individual goals, which gives people a profound reason to continue even in old age.

This sense of purpose—whether serving others, following a spiritual calling, or contributing to the community—provides motivation and energy to stay active and engaged in life. People with a clear purpose tend to take better care of their health, stay mentally active, and remain socially engaged, which contributes to greater longevity.

In the Blue Zones, the purpose is clearly expressed: in Okinawa, Japan, they call it "ikigai," which means "reason for being," and in Nicoya, Costa Rica, it is the "life plan," a goal that motivates them to stay active and healthy.

Spirituality also has a positive impact on mental health.

Spiritual practices such as meditation and prayer help calm the mind and improve concentration, which contributes to greater mental clarity and better cognitive function over time.

Meditation, for example, has been shown to have neuroprotective effects by increasing brain plasticity and reducing stress levels, which protects the brain from neurodegenerative diseases such as Alzheimer's.

Spirituality also provides a framework for dealing with mental and emotional challenges, allowing people to approach mental health issues from a more balanced and less distressing perspective. This ability to maintain calm and mental clarity through spirituality contributes to greater longevity.

Finally, the connection to something larger than oneself that spirituality offers provides a sense of peace and acceptance that can reduce the fear and anxiety associated with aging and death.

By integrating a broader view of life, many spiritual people develop an accepting attitude toward death, allowing them to experience the aging process with greater serenity and less anxiety.

This calmer and more balanced approach to the life cycle not only improves the quality of life in later life but has also been linked to greater longevity.

Intuitive nutrition and the connection with food.

Intuitive eating is an approach to eating that promotes a conscious connection between the body and food, based on internal hunger and satiety cues rather than rigid external rules or restrictive diets.

This approach, increasingly popular in the health and wellness field, moves away from the idea that certain foods are intrinsically good or bad and focuses on the relationship people have with food.

Intuitive nutrition seeks to restore that natural connection with food, trusting the body's innate ability to regulate eating in a balanced and healthy way, rather than relying on externally imposed eating patterns. Through this approach, people learn to respect their physical and emotional needs, leading to improved physical health as well as mental and emotional well-being.

One of the fundamental principles of intuitive eating is recognizing the body's hunger and satiety cues. Over time, many people lose the ability to properly interpret these cues due to the influence of restrictive diets or social norms about how, when, and how much to eat.

Intuitive eating teaches us how to reconnect with these innate cues, encouraging us to eat when we truly feel hungry and stop when we're satisfied, not when we've reached a predetermined amount of food.

This attunement to the body's signals fosters a healthier relationship with food, as it eliminates guilt or obsession with following strict dietary rules and instead promotes a balanced and flexible approach.

The rejection of restrictive diets is another central component of intuitive eating. Traditional diets, often focused on rapid weight loss or the exclusion of certain food groups, can cause a disconnect with the body's signals and lead to a conflicted relationship with food.

Furthermore, restrictive diets often have a counterproductive effect, as they can lead to a dysfunctional relationship with food, marked by episodes of severe restriction followed by binges or feelings of guilt.

Intuitive eating, on the other hand, promotes unrestricted eating where all foods have a place and flexibility is encouraged. By letting go of strict rules, people are able to regain confidence in their ability to choose foods that provide satisfaction and nourishment, without resorting to extreme eating behaviors.

Another important aspect of intuitive eating is the focus on enjoyment and satisfaction in eating. Unlike restrictive diets that often eliminate the pleasure of eating, intuitive eating encourages people to fully enjoy their meals, from food selection to the moment they eat.

It's about paying attention to how food feels in the body and what kind of satisfaction it provides, both physically and emotionally. By enjoying the process of eating, people not only have a more positive experience with food, but they're also less likely to overeat, as they're more in tune with their satiety levels. This approach reduces emotional or impulsive eating patterns and promotes a more mindful relationship with food.

An emotional connection with food is also a key element of intuitive eating. Many people turn to food as a way to cope with difficult emotions, such as stress, sadness, or anxiety.

While it's natural for food to provide comfort in certain moments, intuitive eating encourages people to identify and address the underlying emotions that may be driving emotional eating. Rather than using food as the sole source of comfort, people are encouraged to find other healthy ways to cope with their emotions, such as meditation, physical activity, or talking with loved ones.

This process of emotional introspection helps people avoid overusing food as a coping mechanism, which in turn improves both physical health and mental well-being.

Body acceptance is another essential principle of intuitive eating. This approach promotes the idea that a person's worth is not dependent on their weight or physical appearance, and seeks to challenge the diet culture that imposes unrealistic beauty standards.

Rather than focusing on achieving a specific weight, intuitive eating focuses on holistic well-being, which includes physical, emotional, and mental health. This approach fosters greater self-esteem and respect for the body, allowing people to enjoy food without guilt or shame. By accepting the body as it is, the pressure to meet unrealistic ideals is reduced and a more positive and respectful relationship with food and oneself is fostered.

Furthermore, mindful eating is a powerful tool within intuitive nutrition. Mindful eating involves being fully present during the eating experience, paying attention to the flavors, textures, smells, and physical sensations each food produces.

This mindful approach allows people to more fully enjoy their meals while helping them recognize when they are satisfied, reducing the tendency to overeat. Mindful eating also fosters a greater connection with food, allowing for a deeper appreciation of its nutritional value and emotional satisfaction.

Practicing mindful eating helps prevent impulsive or inertial eating and instead fosters a richer and more rewarding eating experience.

An additional aspect of intuitive eating is the elimination of guilt around food. Modern society often promotes the idea that certain foods are "good" or "bad," leading to feelings of guilt or shame when consuming certain types of foods. Intuitive eating challenges this mentality by teaching that all foods can be part of a healthy diet, as long as they are eaten in moderation and in response to the body's hunger and fullness cues.

By letting go of guilt around food, people can enjoy their favorite foods without experiencing negative emotions, which in turn fosters a more balanced and healthy relationship with food.

Ultimately, intuitive eating not only promotes individual health but also fosters a deeper connection with the environment and the origin of their food. This approach encourages people to be more aware of where their food comes from, how it is grown, and how it impacts the environment.

Intuitive eating often encourages choosing fresh, local, and seasonal foods, which not only benefits personal health but also promotes more sustainable eating practices. This connection with food, beyond its nutritional value, invites people to reflect on how their food choices impact the world around them, promoting a more conscious and respectful relationship with natural resources.

The balance between work, life and rest

Work-life balance is a key concept for maintaining a healthy, productive, and fulfilling life. In an increasingly fast-paced and demanding world, finding the right balance between work responsibilities, personal activities, and time for rest has become a constant challenge for many people.

A lack of this balance can lead to high levels of stress, burnout, and an overall decline in well-being, affecting both physical and mental health. However, achieving harmony between these three areas can improve quality of life, increase productivity, and promote greater personal satisfaction.

Work is an essential part of most people's lives, not only because it provides a source of income but also because it often provides a sense of purpose and accomplishment. However, overwork or the inability to disconnect from work responsibilities can lead to burnout, a condition that affects both performance and emotional health.

Burnout is the result of continuous overload, which generates fatigue, lack of motivation, and a negative attitude toward work. To prevent it, it's crucial to establish clear boundaries between work and personal time, allowing for a true disconnect at the end of the workday. This balance not only improves the quality of the work performed but also allows for proper recovery, which increases energy and creativity in the long run.

Rest is a fundamental pillar for achieving work-life balance. Adequate rest isn't limited to sleep alone, although this is essential for the regeneration of the body and mind, but also to taking regular breaks throughout the day to disconnect from work-related stress.

Getting a good night's sleep, generally between seven and nine hours, is crucial for maintaining good physical health, as during sleep the body repairs tissues, consolidates memory, and regulates the immune system.

Lack of sleep or insufficient rest directly affects cognitive ability, concentration, and mood, decreasing productivity and increasing the risk of errors at work. Furthermore, mental rest during the day, such as taking short breaks or practicing digital disconnection, is equally important. These breaks reduce stress and prevent accumulated fatigue, improving overall performance.

One of the biggest challenges in finding a balance between work and rest is the blurred lines between work and personal time, especially with the rise of remote work and technologies that keep us connected 24/7. Constant availability via email, video calls, and messaging apps can cause rest time to become encroached upon by work demands, making it difficult to mentally disconnect.

To counteract this effect, it's necessary to set clear boundaries, such as disabling notifications outside of work hours or creating dedicated workspaces, which helps physically separate work time from personal time. These practices allow you to protect your downtime and fully enjoy your life outside of work.

Personal time, or time for life outside of work, is equally important for achieving a healthy balance. Taking time for pleasurable activities, such as pursuing a hobby, spending time with friends and family, or simply relaxing, is essential for emotional well-being.

This time allows people to disconnect from stress and work responsibilities, recharge, and pursue personal interests. Interpersonal relationships and recreational activities are essential for mental health, as they provide a sense of belonging, satisfaction, and enjoyment, which in turn strengthens emotional resilience and reduces the risk of chronic stress or anxiety.

Work-life balance doesn't mean dividing time equally between these areas, but rather finding a balance that allows you to fulfill your work responsibilities, take care of your personal well-being, and enjoy your free time without feeling overwhelmed or burned out.

This balance is unique to each individual, as it depends on personal circumstances, responsibilities, and individual preferences. However, there are certain universal principles that can guide people in their search for this balance.

First, it's important to establish clear priorities. Knowing which aspects of life are most important at any given moment helps you better allocate your time and energy. At times, work may require more attention, but at other times, personal needs or rest should take priority. Consciously establishing these priorities and adjusting them according to circumstances prevents burnout and ensures you're investing time in what truly matters.

Second, learning to say no to excessive or unnecessary demands is essential to protecting your balance. Overwhelmed by work or personal commitments can lead to fatigue and stress, so it's important to recognize your limits and set boundaries when necessary. Saying no respectfully, both in the workplace and in your personal life, helps you manage your time better and avoid burnout.

Third, time management is essential for achieving a work-life balance. Effective use of time allows you to fulfill work responsibilities without sacrificing personal time or rest. Tools such as daily planning, setting realistic goals, and prioritizing tasks can help increase efficiency and prevent procrastination, reducing the feeling of being constantly busy or stressed.

Finally, it's essential to recognize the importance of self-care. Taking care of yourself involves not only getting adequate rest, but also maintaining a balanced diet, exercising regularly, and seeking out activities that promote emotional well-being, such as meditation or spending time in nature.

Self-care strengthens people's ability to face work and personal challenges with a clear mind and a healthy body. Investing time in physical and emotional well-being isn't a luxury, but a necessity to maintain balance and avoid burnout.

Chapter 8.
Key Factors for Longevity in Balance with Nature

The key factors for longevity in balance with nature are based on the harmonious interaction between humans and the natural environment. Throughout history, communities that have achieved long and healthy lives have demonstrated a deep connection with nature, utilizing natural resources sustainably and maintaining an environmentally friendly lifestyle.

This approach not only promotes a higher quality of life but also fosters physical, mental, and emotional health. In an increasingly urbanized and technologically advanced world, rediscovering the importance of living in harmony with nature can be a key to balanced and meaningful longevity.

One of the key factors for longevity in balance with nature is access to a diet based on fresh, natural foods. Long-lived cultures, such as those living in the Blue Zones, tend to consume fresh, seasonal, and local foods, minimizing dependence on processed and artificial products.

A diet rich in fruits, vegetables, legumes, whole grains, and healthy fats provides the essential nutrients your body needs to stay healthy. Additionally, consuming plant-based products and unprocessed foods reduces your risk of chronic diseases such as diabetes, hypertension, and heart disease, which are often associated with diets high in saturated fats and refined sugars.

This type of diet, which comes directly from nature, not only promotes health but also reduces environmental impact by reducing the carbon footprint and intensive use of resources.

Another key factor is natural and consistent physical activity, which is deeply connected to the environment. Long-lived people tend to lead physically active lives, not necessarily through structured gym workouts, but through everyday activities such as walking, working in the fields or gardens, and performing manual labor.

These activities not only keep the body moving, strengthening muscles and the cardiovascular system, but also allow for a direct connection with nature.

Walking on nature trails, gardening, or simply being outdoors promotes a greater sense of well-being and reduces stress. Regular interaction with nature improves mental health, as spending time in natural environments has been shown to lower cortisol levels and improve mood.

Stress management is another key factor for longevity in balance with nature. People who live in harmony with the natural environment tend to have a healthier relationship with time, work, and rest. In many long-lived communities, such as Ikaria, Greece, life moves at a slower pace, where naps and adequate rest are an important part of the day.

Frequent contact with nature provides a peaceful and tranquil environment that helps reduce chronic stress, one of the leading causes of cardiovascular disease and mental health problems. The practice of meditation, contemplation, and observation of nature are tools that many cultures have used for centuries to promote mental and emotional well-being.

By integrating nature into their daily lives, people can find deeper emotional balance, which contributes to a longer, healthier life.

Air and water quality also play a crucial role in longevity. Living in a natural environment, away from highly polluted urban centers, allows people to breathe cleaner air and have access to pure, contaminant-free water. Air and water pollution are linked to a range of chronic and degenerative diseases, from respiratory problems to heart disease and cancer.

In long-lived communities, such as those on the Nicoya Peninsula in Costa Rica, access to mineral-rich water and a clean environment contribute to better overall health. The purity of these life-giving elements, sourced directly from nature, strengthens the immune system and protects the body from damage caused by toxins and pollutants present in urban environments.

Regular contact with nature has beneficial effects not only on the body, but also on the mind and spirit. Being surrounded by nature—whether mountains, rivers, forests, or oceans—has a restorative impact on mental health.

Numerous studies have shown that contact with nature reduces levels of anxiety, depression, and stress, while increasing feelings of well-being and happiness. People who live close to nature tend to experience greater life satisfaction, as nature offers a peaceful refuge and an opportunity to disconnect from the hustle and bustle of modern life.

Furthermore, exposure to sunlight, which is abundant in natural environments, is essential for the production of vitamin D, which strengthens bones and the immune system and improves mood. This contact with the natural environment is a constant reminder of the intrinsic connection between human beings and the world around them.

An additional key aspect is sustainability and respect for nature. Long-lived communities tend to have a more sustainable relationship with their environment, using natural resources consciously and avoiding overexploitation. Instead of overconsuming or damaging the environment, these cultures practice sustainable agriculture, responsible fishing, and other activities that protect local ecosystems.

This respect for nature not only ensures that future generations can also enjoy natural resources, but also promotes a more balanced and healthy relationship with the planet. By living sustainably, people can avoid the stress associated with environmental exploitation and contribute to a healthier and more balanced world for all.

Another key factor for longevity in balance with nature is a sense of community. In long-lived cultures, community

life and social support are fundamental. These communities are often strongly connected, with members working
together in activities related to the land, agriculture, or
fishing. This collaboration and strong sense of belonging
not only foster healthy interpersonal relationships but
also strengthen emotional well-being.

People who feel supported by their community are less
likely to suffer from loneliness and depression, factors that
can shorten lifespans. Furthermore, community life promotes greater cooperation in protecting the natural environment, as resources are managed jointly and sustainably for the common good.

Finally, spirituality connected to nature is another factor
that contributes to longevity in balance with the natural
environment. Many long-lived cultures, such as those of
Okinawa and Nicoya, maintain a strong spiritual connection with nature, viewing the natural world not only as a
resource, but as something sacred and worthy of respect.

This spirituality, based on respect for life and the environment, promotes a more balanced and conscious life. Spiritual practices that involve nature, such as outdoor meditation or harvest gratitude rituals, strengthen the bond between humans and the planet, which in turn promotes a
more balanced mindset and greater longevity.

In conclusion, key factors for longevity in balance with nature include a diet based on fresh, natural foods, regular
physical activity in natural settings, effective stress management through contact with nature, access to clean air

and water, sustainability, and a deep sense of community and spirituality connected to one's environment.

This holistic approach not only improves physical health but also promotes mental and emotional well-being, creating a longer, more balanced life in harmony with the planet. Nature, when consciously integrated into daily life, becomes a source of health, longevity, and inner balance.

The importance of living close to nature

Living close to nature has a profound and positive impact on people's physical, mental, and emotional health. In an increasingly urbanized and digitalized world, proximity to the natural environment provides a necessary counterbalance that promotes overall well-being and improves quality of life.

Several studies have shown that people who live in natural environments, such as rural areas, forested areas, or near bodies of water, enjoy greater health benefits compared to those who live in densely populated urban areas.

Nature not only provides a healthier environment from an environmental perspective, but also offers opportunities for physical activity, mental rest, and spiritual connection—essential elements for a balanced and long life.

One of the main benefits of living close to nature is access to a cleaner environment. In rural and natural areas, air pollution levels are often considerably lower than in cities, where vehicle emissions and industrial activity affect air quality.

Breathing clean air is essential for maintaining good lung and cardiovascular health, as prolonged exposure to pollution has been linked to respiratory diseases, such as asthma and chronic bronchitis, as well as heart problems. Furthermore, natural areas provide access to purer water free of chemical contaminants, which contributes to improved overall health.

The natural environment acts as a purifying system, where trees, rivers, and soil filter the air and water, providing a healthier and safer environment.

Stress reduction is another key benefit of living close to nature. Natural environments have a restorative effect on the mind, helping to reduce anxiety and chronic stress. Studies have shown that spending time in nature decreases levels of cortisol, the stress hormone, which improves mood and promotes a greater sense of calm.

The simple act of walking through a forest, gazing at the sea, or listening to the sounds of birds can have an immediate impact on stress reduction, contributing to better mental health. Living close to nature provides easy access to these restorative spaces, allowing people to disconnect from the pressures of everyday life and rejuvenate both mentally and emotionally.

This direct connection with nature acts as a natural form of stress detox, preventing long-term mental health problems such as depression and anxiety.

Access to natural physical activity

This is another benefit of living close to nature. People who live in rural or natural environments tend to engage in more varied and frequent physical activities than those who live in cities.

Opportunities to walk, run, bike, swim, or garden are abundant in natural areas, encouraging an active and healthy lifestyle. Regular physical activity is essential for maintaining good health, as it helps prevent chronic diseases such as obesity, type 2 diabetes, and heart disease.

Furthermore, physical activity in nature not only exercises the body but also provides mental benefits, as being outdoors has a positive effect on mood and motivation. People who live close to nature often find it easier to integrate exercise into their daily lives, which contributes to greater longevity and overall well-being.

Improvement in mental health

It's one of the most important benefits of living close to nature. Various studies have shown that people who live in natural environments experience fewer symptoms of depression, anxiety, and other mental disorders compared to those who live in urban areas.

Regular contact with nature has a therapeutic effect on the brain, promoting relaxation and mental clarity. Furthermore, exposure to natural light and the more pronounced day-night cycles in rural areas help regulate circadian rhythms, improving sleep quality, an essential factor for mental health.

Getting a good night's sleep and restful sleep are essential for maintaining emotional balance and preventing problems such as insomnia and mental exhaustion. In short, living close to nature provides a more favorable environment for mental health, reducing the risk of psychological disorders and promoting greater emotional resilience.

Living close to nature

In addition to the physical and mental benefits, living close to nature also promotes a greater spiritual and emotional connection with one's surroundings. Nature has the ability to inspire a sense of wonder, gratitude, and belonging, which can have a profound impact on emotional and spiritual well-being.

People who live close to nature often develop a more conscious and respectful relationship with their surroundings, which provides them with a sense of purpose and connection to something greater than themselves. This spiritual connection with nature fosters a sense of inner peace, balance, and life satisfaction.

Furthermore, nature offers a space for reflection and contemplation, allowing people to find a peaceful refuge amidst the demands of daily life.

Access to healthier and more sustainable food

This is another important factor that highlights the importance of living close to nature. In many rural or natural areas, people have direct access to fresh, locally sourced foods, such as fruits, vegetables, legumes, and produce. This not only promotes a more balanced and nutrient-dense diet, but also encourages more sustainable eating, minimizing the environmental impact associated with food transportation and processing.

Rural communities often practice local and sustainable agriculture, ensuring a constant supply of healthy, fresh food. Growing one's own food, such as a home garden, not only provides fresh produce but also promotes a closer connection with nature's cycles and food production processes.

Another key aspect is protection against the negative effects of urbanization and modern life. Living in densely populated urban areas often exposes people to higher levels of pollution, noise, and stress.

Large cities can create a feeling of sensory and mental overload, which increases the risk of chronic stress and modern lifestyle-related illnesses. In contrast, people who live close to nature are protected from many of these factors, which contributes to a greater sense of well-being.

The tranquility of natural surroundings, noise reduction, and proximity to open, green spaces provide a more favorable environment for overall health.

Finally, living close to nature also fosters greater environmental awareness. People who are more connected to nature are often more aware of the need to protect the environment and practice sustainability. This not only benefits the individual but also promotes a more respectful and responsible relationship with the planet.

By living in a natural environment, people tend to develop a greater appreciation for natural resources and adopt more sustainable practices, such as recycling, water conservation, and reducing energy consumption.

This environmental awareness not only improves the quality of life for people who live close to nature, but also contributes to the preservation of ecosystems for future generations.

The impact of clean air and sunlight on longevity

This is a fundamental topic in the study of how the natural environment influences long-term health and well-being. These two essential elements of nature, clean air and sunlight, have profound effects on the human body, and their presence or absence can make a significant difference in the quality of life and its length.

Throughout history, people who have lived in areas with access to clean air and adequate sunlight have demonstrated better physical and mental health, which has contributed to greater longevity.

In a world where urban areas are increasingly polluted and outdoor time is decreasing, understanding the importance of these natural factors is crucial to promoting a healthy lifestyle and prolonging life.

One of the main effects of clean air is its ability to improve respiratory and cardiovascular health. Clean air, free of pollutants such as carbon dioxide, carbon monoxide, fine particles, and other harmful chemicals, allows the lungs to function optimally. Chronically breathing polluted air is linked to a number of health problems, including asthma, chronic lung disease, bronchitis, and lung cancer.

Furthermore, air pollution is associated with an increased risk of cardiovascular diseases, such as hypertension and heart attacks, as polluting particles can enter the bloodstream and damage blood vessels. In contrast, people who live in areas with clean, fresh air, such as rural or mountainous areas, are less likely to develop these health conditions, which contributes to greater longevity.

Clean air also has a positive impact on the immune system. Pollutants in urban air not only affect the lungs and heart, but can also weaken the immune system, making it more vulnerable to infections and chronic diseases.

Breathing fresh, clean air, on the other hand, allows the immune system to function more efficiently, protecting the body from infections and strengthening its natural defenses. This effect is particularly important for older people, since as we age, the immune system tends to weaken.

Continued exposure to a pollutant-free environment can help reduce the risk of disease and promote a longer, healthier life.

In addition, clean air contributes to improved mental well-being. Air pollution not only affects the physical body but also negatively impacts mental health. Studies have shown that exposure to high levels of air pollution is linked to an increase in anxiety, depression, and other mental disorders.

Polluted air can negatively affect the brain, reducing adequate oxygenation and increasing oxidative stress, which impairs mood and cognitive function. In contrast, clean, fresh air, especially when combined with nature, has a calming and restorative effect on the mind, helping to reduce stress and anxiety.

This is essential for healthy longevity, as mental well-being is just as important as physical well-being for a full and satisfying life.

As for sunlight, its role in longevity is equally crucial. Moderate exposure to sunlight is essential for the production of vitamin D, a vital vitamin for bone health and immune function. Sunlight activates vitamin D synthesis in the skin, which helps the body absorb calcium, strengthening bones and reducing the risk of diseases such as osteoporosis and fractures, which are common in older people.

Vitamin D deficiency, which is common in those who spend a lot of time indoors or live in areas with little sunlight, has been linked to an increased risk of heart disease, type 2 diabetes, autoimmune diseases, and certain types of cancer. Therefore, ensuring you get enough sunlight is essential for maintaining bone health and preventing chronic diseases that can shorten life.

Sunlight also has a positive impact on mental health. Exposure to sunlight stimulates the production of serotonin, a neurotransmitter that regulates mood and promotes feelings of well-being and happiness.

Lack of sunlight, especially during the winter months or in areas with limited sun exposure, can contribute to the development of mood disorders, such as seasonal depression (seasonal affective disorder or SAD). People who spend more time outdoors, exposed to natural sunlight, tend to experience fewer symptoms of depression and anxiety, which improves their emotional well-being.

Maintaining a positive mood is a crucial component of longevity, as chronic stress and mental disorders are linked to an increased risk of physical illness and a lower quality of life.

Another key benefit of sunlight is its ability to regulate circadian rhythms and improve sleep quality.

Circadian rhythms, the body's natural sleep-wake cycles, are influenced by exposure to sunlight. Natural light helps synchronize the biological clock, regulating sleep patterns and ensuring people get sufficient, restful sleep.

Getting a good night's sleep is essential for longevity, as sleep allows the body to recover and repair tissues, strengthen the immune system, and process cognitive information. Lack of sleep or poor quality sleep has been linked to a number of health problems, including an increased risk of heart disease, diabetes, and cognitive decline.

Sunlight therefore plays an essential role in promoting healthy sleep, which contributes to greater longevity.

The right balance in sun exposure. It's also important. While sunlight has many benefits, it's critical to avoid excessive exposure, which can increase the risk of skin cancer.

Taking steps to protect your skin from ultraviolet (UV) radiation, such as wearing sunscreen and appropriate clothing, allows you to enjoy the benefits of sunlight without the associated risks. Moderate sun exposure, at controlled times, maximizes the positive effects without compromising skin health.

Furthermore, both fresh air and sunlight encourage outdoor physical activity, which in turn improves overall health and longevity. People who live in natural environments or spend more time outdoors tend to be more physically active, whether through walking, running, playing sports, or simply enjoying nature.

Regular physical activity is one of the pillars of a long and healthy life, as it improves cardiovascular health, strengthens muscles and bones, reduces the risk of chronic diseases, and improves mental well-being.

Fresh air and sunlight make these activities more enjoyable, motivating people to stay active and enjoy the physical and mental benefits of being outdoors.

Local and seasonal food

Local and seasonal eating is a nutritional approach based on consuming foods produced close to where we live and available at their peak natural growth. This approach, which has gained relevance in recent years, offers multiple benefits for both human health and the environment, promoting a more direct connection with nature and sustainability.

Local and seasonal foods are not only fresher and more nutritious, but they also help reduce the carbon footprint associated with food transportation and boost the local economy.

One of the main benefits of consuming local foods is that these products are usually fresher and more nutritious. Foods grown close to where they are consumed don't need to travel long distances or be stored for long periods of time, meaning they reach our tables at their peak ripeness. This not only improves the flavor but also maximizes the content of nutrients, such as vitamins and minerals.

Many studies have shown that foods lose nutrients as time passes since they are harvested, so the closer they are to their source, the greater their nutritional value.

Furthermore, by choosing locally sourced foods, we support local producers and farmers, which strengthens regional economies and promotes greater food self-sufficiency. Buying local products allows small and medium-sized farms to remain in business, preserving biodiversity and traditional agricultural practices that are often lost in industrial production.

These producers often use more sustainable farming methods, which contributes to soil conservation and reduces the use of pesticides and chemical fertilizers that can harm the environment.

Seasonal eating also has a positive impact on health. Seasonal foods are naturally at their best nutritionally and flavorfully because they are grown in the right conditions, without the need for greenhouses or artificial techniques that alter their growth cycle.

For example, fruits like strawberries in the summer or oranges in the winter are at their peak ripeness and flavor when consumed in their corresponding season. Furthermore, the seasonal cycle of foods provides us with natural nutritional variety throughout the year, which promotes a balanced diet rich in essential nutrients that vary according to the season.

Another important benefit of consuming seasonal foods is that they tend to be more affordable. Due to the abundance of produce at its natural harvest time, the cost of seasonal foods is typically lower compared to foods produced out of season and requiring more resources and technology to grow.

This makes local and seasonal food more accessible to a greater number of people, allowing for a healthy diet without having to spend large sums of money.

From an environmental perspective, eating local and seasonal foods significantly reduces the carbon footprint associated with food transportation and storage.

Produce grown far from its intended location requires lengthy transportation, storage, and refrigeration processes, which increases greenhouse gas emissions. By consuming local and seasonal produce, we reduce the need for long-distance transportation and the use of fossil fuels, thereby contributing to the fight against climate change.

Additionally, by eating seasonal foods, you reduce your dependence on intensive, energy-intensive farming practices that grow crops outside their natural cycle.

Another positive aspect of eating local and seasonal food is that it fosters a greater connection with nature and the earth's natural cycles. By consuming seasonal produce, people become more aware of agricultural cycles and climatic conditions, which promotes a more harmonious relationship with the natural environment.

This approach reminds us of the importance of respecting nature's rhythms and living sustainably in tune with the resources it offers us. Furthermore, getting to know local farmers and understanding the process behind food production fosters a greater appreciation and respect for what we eat.

Additionally, local and seasonal eating promotes dietary diversity. As we follow seasonal cycles, our diet becomes more varied, incorporating different foods throughout the year.

Instead of consuming the same products all the time, this approach encourages us to enjoy a wide range of fruits, vegetables, and other foods that provide different nutrients and flavors depending on the season.

This dietary diversity is not only beneficial for human health, by ensuring a varied intake of vitamins and minerals, but also for the environment, as it supports agricultural biodiversity and reduces dependence on intensive monocultures.

Finally, local and seasonal food can also have a positive impact on culture and food traditions. By consuming foods typical of the region and in their natural season, local culinary customs are preserved and a greater appreciation for traditional dishes is fostered.

Recipes passed down from generation to generation are often tied to the produce harvested in a specific region during a particular time of year. Maintaining these practices not only supports the local economy but also protects cultural heritage and promotes a richer, more meaningful relationship with food.

The connection between sustainable living and long-term health

The connection between sustainable living and long-term health is increasingly evident in a world where consumer habits and lifestyles have a direct impact on both the environment and personal well-being.

Living sustainably not only benefits the planet by reducing our ecological footprint, but also promotes better physical, mental, and emotional health, which can contribute to greater longevity.

This approach involves adopting practices that respect natural resources, minimize waste, and promote a more conscious and balanced lifestyle. By doing so, people experience an improvement in their quality of life and a greater likelihood of enjoying a long and healthy life.

One of the clearest ways sustainable living supports long-term health is through mindful eating. Choosing a diet based on local, seasonal, and minimally processed foods not only reduces environmental impact but also promotes better nutrition.

Fresh, unprocessed foods contain more essential nutrients, such as vitamins, minerals, and antioxidants, which are key to preventing chronic diseases like type 2 diabetes, heart disease, and certain types of cancer. Furthermore, reducing consumption of ultra-processed and animal-based products reduces the risk of health problems related to an unbalanced diet, such as obesity, high cholesterol, and hypertension.

People who adopt a sustainable diet often enjoy improved digestive health, more energy, and greater longevity.

Waste reduction is another fundamental aspect of sustainable living that also benefits health. Minimizing waste, whether through recycling, reusing materials, or conscious shopping, reduces exposure to chemicals and pollutants found in many consumer products.

For example, reducing plastic use and opting for natural, reusable materials helps reduce exposure to microplastics and toxins that can affect long-term health. Furthermore, living more sustainably also means being more conscious of the products we use in our daily environment, from cleaning products to cosmetics, choosing options that are safer and less harmful to the body.

This reduction in exposure to toxic substances contributes to disease prevention and, therefore, a longer, healthier life.

Another important link between sustainable living and long-term health is the regular physical activity that often accompanies a more conscious lifestyle. People who choose a more sustainable lifestyle tend to incorporate activities such as walking, cycling, or gardening into their daily routine, rather than relying on motorized vehicles to get around.

These forms of physical activity not only reduce carbon emissions but also encourage a more active lifestyle, which is essential for cardiovascular health, mobility, and mental well-being. Staying physically active regularly helps prevent chronic diseases, improve physical endurance, and increase quality of life—key factors in longevity.

Connection with nature is another central aspect of sustainable living that directly impacts health and longevity. Living in a way that is closer to and more respectful of the natural environment encourages outdoor activities, which provides multiple benefits for physical and mental health. Spending time in nature reduces stress, improves mood, and strengthens the immune system.

Furthermore, exposure to sunlight is essential for the production of vitamin D, which helps maintain strong bones and prevent age-related diseases such as osteoporosis. People who live in harmony with nature tend to enjoy a greater sense of well-being, which contributes to healthy aging.

Stress management is another significant benefit of sustainable living. By adopting a simpler, more conscious lifestyle, people often experience less pressure and anxiety related to overconsumption and a fast-paced lifestyle.

Sustainable practices, such as voluntary simplicity, minimalism, and connection with the natural environment, promote a more balanced mindset and better management of expectations and stress. This is crucial, as chronic stress is linked to a range of health problems, including heart disease, depression, and sleep disorders, which can shorten lifespans. People who manage to reduce stress through sustainable practices are more likely to enjoy longer, better-quality lives.

Emotional sustainability also plays a role in the connection between sustainable living and long-term health. People who adopt a sustainable approach often develop deeper and more meaningful relationships, as they value quality time with family and friends over consumerism or material possessions.

This focus on interpersonal relationships and community life helps create an emotional support network that is essential for mental well-being. Strong social connections are linked to increased longevity, as they reduce loneliness and isolation, factors that can contribute to physical and mental decline over time.

A focus on sustainability also fosters a greater sense of purpose and responsibility, which is essential for a long and fulfilling life. Living sustainably involves being more mindful of daily decisions and their impact on the world, which creates a sense of purpose and satisfaction.

People who feel their actions are aligned with their values and that they are positively contributing to the well-being of the planet and future generations tend to experience greater life satisfaction. This sense of purpose is directly linked to greater longevity, as people with a clear purpose tend to take better care of their health and remain more active and engaged.

Finally, sustainable living also contributes to the prevention of global diseases related to environmental degradation. Air, water, and soil pollution, as well as biodiversity loss and climate change, have direct effects on human health.

Adopting sustainable practices, such as reducing energy consumption, opting for renewable energy, consuming local and seasonal products, and reducing the use of plastics and chemicals, helps mitigate these problems and, therefore, protects both individual health and that of global communities.

By reducing pollution and protecting natural resources, we create healthier environments that promote longevity for the general population.

Chapter 9.
Living Beyond 100: The Blue Zones Model

It's a concept that explores how certain communities around the world have managed to live significantly longer and with a better quality of life. These areas, known as Blue Zones, are characterized by a high concentration of centenarians, people who live more than 100 years.

Blue Zones are found in various parts of the world, including Okinawa (Japan), Ikaria (Greece), Sardinia (Italy), the Nicoya Peninsula (Costa Rica), and Loma Linda (California, United States). In these regions, life expectancy is significantly higher than the global average, and what makes this phenomenon even more interesting is that people not only live longer, but also do so in good physical and mental health.

The Blue Zones model is based on a combination of habits and lifestyle factors that, together, contribute to longevity. Although each region has its own culture, geography, and particularities, there are certain common elements that define the way of life in these communities and that can be replicated or adapted to improve the quality of life elsewhere.

These factors include diet, physical activity, social relationships, sense of purpose, and stress management, among others. The Blue Zones study has revealed that longevity is not the result of a single factor, but rather the harmonious interaction of several factors that promote well-being throughout life.

Plant-Based Diet

One of the pillars of the Blue Zones model is a plant-based diet. People living in these regions consume mostly plant-based foods, such as fruits, vegetables, legumes, whole grains, and nuts.

Meat, although not completely excluded, is consumed in moderation, generally in small quantities and on special occasions. This diet, rich in antioxidants, vitamins, and minerals, protects against chronic diseases that commonly affect older adults, such as heart disease, cancer, and diabetes.

In Icaria, Greece, for example, the Mediterranean diet, which includes olive oil, legumes, fresh vegetables, and occasional fish, is key to longevity. This natural and balanced diet not only provides the nutrients necessary for a long and healthy life, but also reduces inflammation and oxidative stress in the body, two factors associated with premature aging.

Moderate and Constant Physical Activity

Another important factor in the Blue Zones model is moderate but consistent physical activity. Unlike modern Western societies, where exercise is viewed as a separate and structured activity, Blue Zone residents integrate physical movement into their daily lives. People walk long distances, work in the fields or gardens, and perform manual tasks that keep their bodies moving naturally.

In Sardinia, Italy, shepherds walk several kilometers a day in mountainous terrain, which helps them maintain excellent cardiovascular and muscular health. The key here isn't extreme exercise, but rather regular, sustained movement throughout the day, which helps keep the body strong, agile, and functional even into old age.

Stress Management

Stress management is also a crucial aspect of the Blue Zone lifestyle. People who live more than 100 years in these regions have developed effective ways to reduce and manage stress, which is a key factor in aging and the development of chronic diseases.

In Okinawa, Japan, there's a practice known as "ikigai," which means "reason for being" or "reason for getting up every morning." Having a clear sense of purpose not only provides motivation and satisfaction, but also helps people cope with life's stress and difficulties in a healthier way.

In Icaria and Sardinia, daily naps and adequate rest are common practices that help reduce levels of cortisol, the stress hormone, protecting the body from the negative effects of chronic stress.

Social Relations and Sense of Community

A sense of community and social relationships play a fundamental role in longevity in Blue Zones. People in these regions tend to live in close-knit communities, where family and social relationships are deep and meaningful.

Mutual support, collaboration, and regular social interaction provide a sense of belonging and emotional security that has a positive impact on mental and physical health.

In Okinawa, the concept of "moai" refers to groups of friends who support each other throughout life, strengthening social ties and reducing feelings of loneliness, a factor that has been linked to a shorter life expectancy.

Sense of Purpose

Another key aspect of the Blue Zones model is a sense of purpose. People who live beyond 100 often have a clear purpose in life, whether it's caring for their families, contributing to the community, or engaging in meaningful activities that bring them personal satisfaction.

In Nicoya, Costa Rica, for example, the "life plan" is a central part of the culture, and older adults remain active and engaged with their surroundings, giving them a reason to stay healthy and energetic. This sense of purpose is crucial for longevity, as people who feel their lives have meaning tend to take better care of their health and stay more physically and mentally active.

Work-Life-Relax Balance

Furthermore, work-life balance is a common characteristic of Blue Zones. People in these communities aren't caught up in the stress of a demanding job or the constant pursuit of material success. Instead, they balance their work responsibilities with time for rest, recreation, and socializing.

This ability to disconnect and enjoy life without rushing contributes to better mental and physical health, as it reduces the risk of burnout and stress-related illnesses.

Respect for the Natural Environment

Finally, respect for the natural environment is also an essential component of the Blue Zones model. These communities tend to live in harmony with nature, respecting natural resources and adopting sustainable practices. Regular contact with nature, whether through agriculture, outdoor work, or simply spending time in natural settings, has a restorative effect on both body and mind.

Exposure to sunlight, fresh air, and the natural environment not only improves physical health but also reduces stress and promotes mental well-being.

In short, the Blue Zones model offers a number of valuable lessons on how to live beyond 100 years of age in good health and well-being. Through a combination of a plant-based diet, regular physical activity, stress management, strong social relationships, a sense of purpose, and a lifestyle in harmony with nature, people in these regions have discovered the secrets of longevity.

Although each Blue Zone has its own unique characteristics, the guiding principles are universal and can be adopted anywhere in the world to improve health, prolong life, and enjoy a full and satisfying old age.

Testimonies from long-lived residents in the blue zones

The testimonies of long-lived individuals in the Blue Zones offer a profound and personal insight into how everyday practices can influence longevity. These individuals, who have lived for over 100 years in regions such as Okinawa, Sardinia, Icaria, Nicoya, and Loma Linda, share valuable lessons about the importance of a balanced life, with habits that promote both physical health and mental and emotional well-being.

Testimony of Misao Okawa (Okinawa, Japan)

Misao Okawa, who lived to the age of 117 in Okinawa, attributed her longevity to a combination of a healthy diet, peace of mind, and moderate activity. "Eating fresh fish, vegetables, and tofu has been part of my daily life. I never rushed through life, and I always found time to be with my family. I think that's the key," she shared in an interview on her 115th birthday.

In Okinawa, the concept of "ikigai" (reason for being) is fundamental. Okawa mentioned that her ikigai was to take care of her grandchildren, which gave her a clear purpose throughout her life. This practice of having a purpose and a reason for getting up every morning is common among centenarians in this region.

Testimony of Antonio Todde (Sardinia, Italy)

Antonio Todde, one of Sardinia's oldest men, lived to 112 and used to say, "I've never been alone. I've worked every day of my life, and I've always had my family by my side." In Sardinia, community life is highly valued, and people maintain strong family and social ties.

Todde worked as a shepherd for much of his life, walking long distances through the Sardinian mountains. His daily physical activity, along with a diet based on local products like sheep's milk cheese and red wine, contributed to his longevity. "Work never harmed me, and I've always eaten what the land gave me," he added, highlighting his connection with nature and local food as key to his long life.

Testimony of Stamatis Moraitis (Ikaria, Greece)

Stamatis Moraitis, a Greek immigrant living in the United States, was diagnosed with cancer in his 60s and given only months to live. He decided to return to his hometown of Ikaria, where, to his surprise, he began to feel better and eventually lived to 102.

"In Icaria, we never look at the clock," Moraitis said. The relaxed lifestyle, which includes daily siestas, a Mediterranean diet based on olive oil, legumes, and fish, and strong social connection, was key to his recovery. Moraitis highlighted the tranquility and sense of community as fundamental to his well-being: "Here, we live as if time were eternal, without worries, surrounded by friends."

Testimony of Panchita Castillo (Nicoya, Costa Rica)

On the Nicoya Peninsula, Costa Rica, Panchita Castillo, who lived past 100, shared that the secret to her longevity was "working the land and having faith in God." Panchita, like many other Nicoya centenarians, maintained an active lifestyle, working in the fields well into old age. Her traditional diet of corn, beans, and fresh fruit, along with the region's calcium- and magnesium-rich water, contributed to her robust health.

Panchita also highlighted the value of family in her life: "My children and grandchildren have always surrounded me, and the love of family has kept me strong." This sense of "life plan," or purpose of staying connected to family and community, is a key characteristic among Nicoya's long-lived residents.

Testimony of Ellsworth Wareham (Loma Linda, United States)

Ellsworth Wareham, a retired surgeon and Seventh-day Adventist from Loma Linda, California, lived to the age of

104. He attributed his longevity to a simple life, a vegetarian diet, and the importance of rest. "I've avoided meat for over 50 years, and my body has responded well to that," Wareham said in one of his interviews.

In addition to his diet, Wareham emphasized the importance of spirituality and rest. As a Seventh-day Adventist, he observed the Sabbath, a weekly day of rest dedicated to reflection and spiritual connection. This day of rest allowed him to better manage stress and maintain mental balance, which he believed was key to living a long and healthy life.

Lessons from the Testimonies

These testimonies highlight some essential elements that are common to all Blue Zones:

Plant-based and local food eating. It's key to the longevity of people living in Blue Zones. Most long-lived individuals in these regions consume diets rich in vegetables, legumes, fruits, and healthy fats like olive oil and nuts.

These foods provide a wealth of essential nutrients, such as antioxidants, vitamins, and fiber, which protect against chronic diseases like heart disease, cancer, and diabetes.

By avoiding ultra-processed foods and limiting meat consumption, long-lived people maintain a balanced and natural diet, which not only promotes a long life but also a better quality of life.

Furthermore, consuming local and seasonal foods ensures that the products are fresh, nutritious, and environmentally friendly.

This diet, combined with an active lifestyle, is essential for physical and mental well-being throughout the years.

Moderate physical activity is an essential component of longevity for people living in Blue Zones. Unlike modern approaches that promote intense, structured exercise, long-lived people integrate movement naturally into their daily lives. Activities such as walking, working in the fields, gardening, or doing housework allow them to stay physically active without the need for strenuous routines.

This consistent, yet moderate, movement helps improve cardiovascular health, maintain muscle strength and flexibility, and prevent health problems associated with a sedentary lifestyle, such as obesity and chronic diseases. The key lies in regularity and connection to daily activities, which not only promote physical health but also offer purpose and a connection with nature. This approach to moderate activity is essential for living longer, healthier, and more fulfilling lives.

Strong social connection is a key factor in the longevity of people in Blue Zones. Deep relationships with family, friends, and the community provide constant emotional support and a sense of belonging that strengthens mental and physical health. Being surrounded by people who provide companionship and assistance in times of need reduces stress and feelings of loneliness, both of which can shorten life expectancy.

Regular social interaction fosters emotional well-being, as people feel they are part of something larger than themselves. This social support not only provides emotional stability but also improves quality of life by promoting collaboration and mutual care.

Close-knit communities help people feel valued, motivated, and secure, which directly contributes to better mental and physical health and a longer, more fulfilling life.

A sense of purpose is a crucial component of longevity for people in the Blue Zones. Having a clear reason for living, whether through work, family, or faith, gives long-lived individuals a constant motivation that drives them to remain active, engaged, and positive about life. This purpose, known in Okinawa as "ikigai" and in Nicoya as "life plan," provides a structure and sense of direction that influences physical and mental health.

A sense of purpose also helps them cope with aging with greater resilience, make healthy choices, and stay involved in their communities.

People who feel their lives have meaning tend to experience less stress and depression, which in turn reduces the risk of chronic diseases and promotes greater longevity. Maintaining this purpose throughout life is key to living with satisfaction and well-being.

Stress management. It's essential for longevity in the Blue Zones, where long-lived individuals have developed simple but effective practices to manage daily stress. One of the most common ways is regular rest, either through daily naps or a weekly day of spiritual disconnection, like the Sabbath in Loma Linda.

These breaks not only allow the body to rest and recover, but they also reduce levels of cortisol, the stress hormone, which in excess can cause heart disease, hypertension, and cognitive decline.

The ability to disconnect from the fast-paced nature of life and dedicate time to relaxation contributes to greater mental clarity and emotional well-being. This approach helps people stay calm in the face of challenges, improve their physical health, and avoid the burnout associated with chronic stress. Together, these practices promote emotional balance, which fosters longevity and a better quality of life.

These testimonies show that longevity is not only the result of good genes, but also of a balanced lifestyle, connected to nature, people, and oneself.

Blue Zones represent a healthy lifestyle model based on habits that promote longevity and well-being. These enclaves, where life expectancy is significantly higher, offer us valuable lessons on how to improve our quality of life.

By applying Blue Zone principles—such as a plant-based diet, moderate and consistent physical activity, strong social connection, a sense of purpose, and effective stress management—we can increase our chances of living beyond 100.

Adopting a diet rich in natural, local foods, staying active through daily activities, and strengthening our social relationships are simple steps that contribute to a long and healthy life.

Additionally, having a clear purpose and practicing regular rest help reduce stress and improve our mental health. Blue Zones are an example of how small changes in our lifestyle can have a big impact on our longevity.

The values and life principles that promote longevity.

These values are deeply rooted in the practices and habits of the communities living in Blue Zones. These areas are characterized by the presence of people who not only live to more than 100 years, but also do so with a high quality of life, maintaining their physical, mental, and emotional well-being.

The principles these people follow are linked to a balanced and conscious lifestyle, where core values guide their daily decisions. These values not only improve individual health but also promote harmony with the community and the natural environment.

One of the key principles is respect for nature and conscious eating. In the Blue Zones, the diet is based on local, plant-based products, which not only provide the nutrients necessary for health but also respect the natural cycles of the earth. Eating a balanced diet, limiting the consumption of processed foods and meat, is a fundamental value that protects against chronic diseases and promotes longevity.

This respect for nature also extends to a life in harmony with the environment, where people value natural resources and use them sustainably.

Another crucial value is the focus on social relationships and community. People in Blue Zones have strong ties with their families, friends, and neighbors. Social support, collaboration, and regular interaction promote a sense of belonging and emotional security that is essential for a long and healthy life.

This principle of community is a core value in these cultures, as close relationships not only provide companionship but also help reduce stress and foster a positive attitude toward aging.

A sense of purpose is another essential principle that defines the lives of long-lived people. Having a clear reason for living, whether through work, family, or a commitment to community or faith, provides constant motivation to stay active and healthy.

This value, known as "ikigai" in Okinawa and "life plan" in Nicoya, not only gives meaning to daily activities but also helps us face difficulties with greater resilience and determination. People who have a purpose in life tend to take better care of their health, maintain emotional balance, and live with an optimistic attitude.

Stress management. It's another fundamental value that promotes longevity. In Blue Zones, people practice regular rest, whether through naps, spiritual disconnection days, or simply enjoying quiet moments.

The value of calm and mental balance is key to reducing stress levels, which, in excess, can lead to chronic illness. The practice of living a more relaxed life, without rushing and the pressure of a fast-paced lifestyle, allows long-lived people to avoid the emotional and physical wear and tear that chronic stress brings.

Moderation and simplicity are also essential values that promote longevity. In these communities, people tend to live with less, valuing the essentials and avoiding excess. This principle applies not only to food, where portions are usually moderate, but also to the way of life in general.

Simplicity fosters a lifestyle free from unnecessary complications, reducing stress and allowing for a clearer focus on what truly matters, such as health, family, and community.

Finally, a focus on spirituality and faith is a value that also plays an important role in longevity. In some Blue Zones, such as Loma Linda, California, spiritual and religious practices provide a framework for rest, reflection, and self-care.

This value not only fosters inner peace and emotional resilience, but also provides greater perspective in the face of life's challenges, helping people face aging and death with serenity.

Spirituality provides a source of comfort and emotional well-being that is essential to maintaining balanced mental health.

How to adapt blue zone habits to your daily life.

Adapt Blue Zone habits to your daily lifeIt's an excellent way to improve your health and well-being, and possibly increase your longevity. People living in Blue Zones have shown that small lifestyle changes can make a big difference in the quality and length of life. Here are some practical ways to adapt these habits to your daily life:

.

1. Adopt a Plant-Based Diet

One of the key common threads across all Blue Zones is the predominance of a plant-based diet, rich in vegetables, fresh fruits, legumes, nuts, and whole grains. These communities don't follow strict or complicated diets, but rather eat in a simple, natural, and nutritious way.

You can start by making small changes to your daily diet. Incorporate more plant-based foods such as colorful salads, soups with lentils or chickpeas, brown rice dishes with vegetables, or smoothies with fruits and leafy greens. Legumes such as lentils, beans, and chickpeas are an excellent source of plant-based protein, fiber, and essential minerals, which help maintain gut health, control blood sugar, and lower cholesterol.

Reduce consumption of red meat and ultra-processed foods, which are often loaded with saturated fats, sugars, and preservatives.

In Blue Zones, meat consumption is sporadic and usually reserved for special occasions. Instead, they prioritize fresh, local, and seasonal foods.

Furthermore, this type of diet helps prevent chronic diseases such as hypertension, type 2 diabetes, cardiovascular disease, and some types of cancer. It also improves intestinal transit, strengthens the immune system, and gives you more energy for your daily life.

Adopting a plant-based diet doesn't mean completely eliminating other foods, but rather balancing your diet by emphasizing natural and nutritious options, just like the world's longest-lived people do. Your body, mind, and overall well-being will thank you for it.

2. Move Naturally: Activate Your Body Without Extreme Effort

Contrary to popular belief, you don't need to join a gym or do intense workouts every day to be physically fit. In Blue Zones, long-lived people stay naturally active, integrating movement into their daily lives spontaneously, fluidly, and consistently.

Instead of exercising out of obligation, they move as part of their daily routine: they walk long distances, farm, tend to their gardens, do housework, cook, clean, walk to the market, or use bicycles as a means of transportation. This type of moderate but consistent movement keeps their bodies strong, agile, and healthy throughout their lives.

You too can adopt this principle by starting to incorporate more conscious movement into your daily routine:

- Take the stairs instead of the elevator.

- Walk or bike to work or shopping.

- Spend time caring for plants, fixing up your home, or just taking a walk outdoors.

- Take active breaks if you work sitting for many hours.

- Organize walks with friends or family to socialize while you move.

This type of activity not only improves cardiovascular health, muscle strength, and flexibility, but also helps reduce stress, improve mood, and keep your mind active. The most important thing is to keep moving regularly, without the need for strenuous routines or external pressures.

The secret is to make movement a natural and pleasurable part of your lifestyle, just as the inhabitants of the Blue Zones do. Your body doesn't need perfection, it needs consistency. Move with joy, with purpose, and you'll see how your energy and well-being transform.

3. Develop a Strong Social Connection: Cultivate Bonds that Nourish Your Life

One of the most powerful keys to a long and happy life, observed in all Blue Zones, is the importance of deep and meaningful human relationships. Long-lived people take care not only of their bodies but also of their hearts through the bonds they build with others.

Fostering strong relationships with family, friends, and community isn't a luxury; it's a vital necessity. It's proven that those who have a strong emotional support network have lower stress levels, better mental health, a lower likelihood of heart disease, and greater resilience in the face of life's challenges.

You can start by spending quality time with those you love: share a meal without distractions, make a call to check in on someone, plan simple get-togethers like walks, board games, or relaxed conversations. It's not the activity that matters, but the presence and genuine connection.

You can also expand your social circle by participating in groups with common interests: workshops, sports activities, volunteer opportunities, or community gatherings. These spaces foster a sense of belonging and connect you with people who can enrich your life.

In the Blue Zones, it's common to see multigenerational families living together or very close to each other, neighbors looking out for each other, and support groups like the "moai" in Okinawa, where people support each other throughout their lives.

Strong social connections act as an emotional support network, reducing isolation, anxiety, and depression. They also provide motivation, companionship, and joy—essential elements for a fulfilling and purposeful life.

Remember: the quality of your relationships directly influences the quality of your life. Don't underestimate the power of a heartfelt conversation, a shared laugh, or a helping hand. Cultivate your relationships like a garden: with time, dedication, and love.

4. Find Your Life Purpose: Live with Meaning Every Day

One of the most powerful pillars shared by long-lived people in the Blue Zones is having a clear and meaningful purpose in life. It's not just about living a long life, but about living meaningfully, with a reason to get up every morning and contribute to the world around us.

In Okinawa, this concept is known as "ikigai," and in Nicoya, it's called "life plan." In both cases, it refers to that inner force that drives you, gives you direction, and makes your existence meaningful beyond daily routines. Having a purpose not only strengthens the spirit, but has also been directly linked to better health, greater longevity, a lower incidence of mental illness, and a stronger immune system.

What inspires you? What moves you? What makes you feel like your life has meaning? Purpose can take many forms: caring for your family, teaching, creating art, gardening, serving your community, learning something new, helping others, or following a personal passion. It doesn't have to be something grand or public; the important thing is that it's authentic to you.

Discovering and living your purpose has multiple benefits:

It gives you daily motivation, and helps you overcome difficult times.

Promote healthy habits, because you take better care of yourself when you know your life has value.

Strengthen your self-esteem, and connects you with others from a place of contribution.

It keeps you mentally and emotionally active, which is essential for overall well-being.

If you're still not clear about your purpose, don't worry. Searching is also part of the journey. You can start by asking yourself questions like:

- What activities make me lose track of time?

- What would I like to contribute to the world?

- What brings me deep joy or lasting satisfaction?

You can also write, talk to people who inspire you, or try new experiences until you find what resonates with you.

Living with purpose transforms ordinary life into an extraordinary experience.It doesn't just add years to your life, it adds life to your years. As the Blue Zones demonstrate, a sense of purpose isn't a spiritual luxury; it's a vital necessity.

5. Manage Stress Regularly: Give Your Mind and Body Breaks

Although stress is an inevitable part of life, managing it effectively is one of the most important keys to a long and healthy life, as demonstrated by the long-lived communities in the Blue Zones. It's not that these people don't experience stress, but rather that they have developed healthy and consistent ways to release it before it affects their well-being.

In places like Okinawa, Nicoya, and Loma Linda, stress management is part of the lifestyle, not as a reaction, but as a conscious, daily preventive measure. This allows the body and mind time to rest, regenerate, and heal.

How can you do this in your daily life?

Include intentional breaks throughout the day. You don't have to wait until you're exhausted to rest. You can take a short nap, close your eyes for a few minutes, breathe deeply, or simply disconnect from your devices.

Practice relaxing activities. Reading, gardening, a walk in nature, soft music, or even a relaxing shower can become wellness rituals that calm your nervous system.

Incorporates mindfulness practices. Techniques such as meditation, yoga, conscious breathing, and prayer have been shown to reduce cortisol (the stress hormone), improve mental clarity, and promote states of inner peace.

Come back to the present moment. Stress often comes from thinking too much about the future or about things you can't control. Learning to live in the present with acceptance and gratitude is a powerful healing tool.

Connect with what you love. Spending time with loved ones, laughing, caring for a plant, or preparing a loving meal are also ways to release accumulated tension.

Chronic stress is associated with numerous illnesses, including high blood pressure, heart disease, anxiety, depression, and a weakened immune system. Therefore, Blue Zones prioritize rest, contemplation, and emotional balance as fundamental health habits.

Giving yourself spaces of calm is not wasting time, it's protecting your life. Learning to stop, breathe, and recharge not only improves your immediate well-being, but also allows you to live longer and more fully.

6. Live Moderately and Simply: Find Fulfillment in the Essential

A deeply rooted characteristic of Blue Zones is a simple, balanced, and excess-free life. Far from the consumerism and accelerated pace that dominates many modern societies, these long-lived communities teach us that living well doesn't mean having more, but rather needing less.

Moderation is a philosophy of life that applies to all areas: from nutrition to time management, from material possessions to personal relationships. Long-lived people don't seek to fill their lives with things, but rather with meaning, connection, and authentic well-being.

How can you apply this wisdom in your daily life?

Simplify your diet: Eat when you're hungry, stop when you're full. Practice moderation in portions (like the "Hara Hachi Bu" principle in Okinawa: eat until you're 80% full). Choose natural, local, and fresh foods, without the need to complicate things with strict diets or fads.

Detach yourself from the unnecessary: Live with what you really need. Go through your belongings and ask yourself what things bring you real value. Decluttering your surroundings also frees your mind and reduces stress, allowing you to focus on what's important.

Slow down your pace of life: You don't need to be always busy to be productive. Learning to say "no," resting without guilt, and prioritizing what truly matters will help you maintain your energy, your mental health, and your inner balance.

Avoid emotional excess: Live your emotions authentically, but without allowing unnecessary drama or negativity to drag you down. Practicing calm, gratitude, and acceptance is part of a simple and healthy life.

Value the essential: Appreciate the little things: a heartfelt conversation, a home-cooked meal, the sound of the wind, or the warmth of the sun on your skin. Lasting happiness isn't found in luxuries, but in the ability to enjoy what you already have.

Living moderately and simply connects you with your essence, reduces stress, improves your mental health, and strengthens your emotional well-being. It's a conscious way to live in harmony with yourself, others, and your environment.

Remember: In the Blue Zones, longevity doesn't come from having more, but from living better, with less, and with greater purpose. In that simplicity lies the true richness of a full life.

7. Connect with Nature: Return to the Rhythm that Nourishes Your Body and Soul

One of the most harmonious and constant elements in the lives of long-lived people in Blue Zones is their deep connection with nature. Whether working the land, walking along rural trails, breathing the fresh country air, or simply gazing at the sunset sky, these people live in harmony with their natural surroundings, and this is directly reflected in their physical, emotional, and spiritual health.

In a world increasingly dominated by screens, noise, asphalt, and haste, reconnecting with nature is not only an act of rest, but an act of healing.

How can you reconnect with nature in your daily life?

Go for a walk outdoors whenever you can. Whether it's in a nearby park, on a beach, in the countryside, or on a mountain, walking among trees or under the open sky helps you clear your mind, reduce stress, and improve your mood.

Grow something living. Having a small vegetable garden, caring for potted plants, or participating in gardening activities connects you directly to the natural cycles of life, fosters patience, and brings satisfaction.

Disconnect from the digital world to reconnect with yourself. Taking a few minutes each day to observe the sky, listen to birdsong, feel the wind, or walk barefoot on the grass can renew your energy in surprising ways.

Do outdoor activities in company. Sharing moments in nature with family or friends not only strengthens social bonds, but also promotes physical activity, laughter, and vitality.

Appreciate natural beauty with all your senses.

Stop to smell a flower, touch the bark of a tree, contemplate the movement of the leaves, or feel the warmth of the sun. Nature teaches us to be present, to breathe calmly, and to live with gratitude.

Numerous studies support what Blue Zones already practice: contact with nature lowers blood pressure, improves the immune system, decreases cortisol (stress) levels, and strengthens mental health. It also reminds us that we are part of a larger whole and that living in balance with our surroundings is key to our fulfillment.

Connecting with nature does not require long trips or excessive time, just a willingness to return to the essential, to what has always been there for you: the natural world that surrounds you and sustains you.

8. Spend Time on Spirituality or Reflection:

Nourish Your Soul to Live with Peace and Purpose. Across all Blue Zones around the world, a common and powerful pattern has been observed: long-lived people regularly dedicate time to spirituality, faith, or deep reflection.

This practice not only provides them with comfort and meaning, but has also been associated with better emotional health, lower stress, greater resilience, and a more positive attitude toward life and death.

Spirituality, in this context, is not limited to a specific religion, but encompasses any form of connection with something greater than oneself. It can include religious faith, meditation, contemplation of nature, daily gratitude, or simply the act of remaining silent and listening to one's heart.

How can you incorporate this principle into your life?

Set aside a time of day for introspection.

Begin or end your day with a few minutes of silence, deep breathing, prayer, or meditation. This small habit can transform your mental and emotional state.

Write down your thoughts or thanks. Keeping a spiritual or gratitude journal helps you recognize the positive in your life, process emotions, and find clarity amidst the chaos.

Participate in activities with spiritual meaning.
Attending a ceremony, a prayer group, guided meditation, or even reading inspirational books can help you reconnect with your values and purpose.

Connect with the present from the soul. Simple moments like watching a sunset, walking in silence, or listening to calming music can also be opportunities to enter a state of deep reflection.

Develop a broader perspective on life. Spirituality helps us accept aging, loss, and challenges as a natural part of the human journey, and gives us the tools to face them with wisdom, acceptance, and serenity.

In Blue Zones, spending time in spirituality has been shown to strengthen mental and emotional health, reduce the risk of depression, improve sleep quality, and foster more empathetic and compassionate relationships. Furthermore, people with an active spiritual life often experience greater personal satisfaction and a more hopeful outlook on the future.

Cultivating your inner world is as important as taking care of your body.

Amidst the noise and demands of the modern world, taking a moment to connect with the transcendent—whatever your path—is an act of self-love.

9. Practice Regular Rest: Renew Yourself to Live Better and Longer

In the Blue Zones, rest is not seen as a luxury or a sign of weakness, but as a fundamental part of the natural cycle of life. Resting throughout the day and sleeping soundly at night is essential for physical, mental, and emotional regeneration. It is during rest that the body heals, the mind clears, and emotions are balanced.

Long-lived people in these regions tend to lead a more relaxed and conscious lifestyle, where rest is part of their daily routine. Whether it's a nap, a quiet break after lunch, or making sure they get a good night's sleep, they understand that well-being isn't achieved through haste, but through balance.

How can you incorporate regular rest into your lifestyle?

Get enough sleep every night. Try to establish a consistent sleep routine, going to bed and waking up at the same time every day. Sound sleep is key for cell repair, brain function, and a stronger immune system.

Allow yourself short naps if your body needs them. A 20- to 30-minute nap can revitalize you, improve your concentration, and reduce stress levels, especially if you have a busy day.

Listen to your body. If you're feeling fatigued, mentally or emotionally exhausted, don't ignore it. Learn to identify the signs that indicate you need to pause, breathe, and recharge.

Create spaces of calm in your daily routine. Rest isn't just about sleeping. Reading a book, closing your eyes for a few minutes, practicing meditation, or simply enjoying a moment of silence are valid and necessary forms of rest.

Respect your limits without guilt. We live in a culture that glorifies constant productivity, but rest is an essential part of an efficient and healthy life. Rest allows you to perform better, think more clearly, and live more fully.

Adequate rest helps prevent physical and emotional exhaustion, improves cognitive performance, reduces the risk of chronic diseases, and promotes a longer, more balanced life. In the Blue Zones, this understanding translates into healthy longevity, where people reach advanced age with energy, vitality, and mental clarity.

Remember: it's not just about taking breaks, but about giving them a restorative purpose. Honoring your rest cycles is a form of deep self-care that strengthens your body, soothes your mind, and rejuvenates your spirit.

10. Cultivate Gratitude and Optimism: A Positive Attitude that Prolongs and Beautifies Life

One of the most consistent traits shared by people who live longer and with a better quality of life in the Blue Zones is their positive attitude toward life. Maintaining an optimistic mindset, accompanied by a consistent practice of gratitude, not only improves mental and emotional health, but also strengthens the body and prolongs life.

Far from denying difficulties, long-lived people choose to focus their attention on the good, on what they have, on what works, and on what brings them joy.

This way of seeing life allows them to face challenges with greater resilience, maintain more harmonious relationships, and enjoy the small everyday moments more intensely.

How can you begin to cultivate gratitude and optimism in your life?

Do a daily gratitude exercise. Take a few minutes each day to reflect on or write down three things you're grateful for. They can be simple: a smile, a meal, a bird's song, or a meaningful conversation. This habit retrains your mind to focus on the positive.

Reframe your internal dialogue. Learn to replace negative thoughts with more compassionate and constructive ones. Instead of saying, "This is a disaster," you can say, "This is a challenge I'm learning to overcome."

Surround yourself with people who add up. Optimism is also contagious. Share your life with people who inspire you, support you, and help you see the bright side of situations.

Celebrate the small achievements. Be grateful for every step you take, every advancement, every experience that has helped you grow. Valuing your progress strengthens motivation and self-esteem.

Find beauty in the everyday. Look at the world with eyes of wonder, as if each day were a gift. Sometimes a flower, a laugh, or a ray of sunshine can completely transform your mood.

Numerous studies have shown that gratitude lowers cortisol (the stress hormone) levels, improves sleep quality, strengthens the immune system, and reduces symptoms of anxiety and depression. Furthermore, maintaining an optimistic attitude contributes to better cardiovascular health and greater longevity.

Choosing to view life with gratitude and hope is not naivety, it is emotional strength.

It is a conscious decision that transforms your way of living, of relating to yourself and the world.

Live Longer and Better, One Habit at a Time

Adapting Blue Zone habits to your life doesn't require drastic changes or extreme sacrifices. Rather, it's about reconnecting with what's essential, returning to what's natural, to what's human, to what truly nourishes the body, mind, and soul.

Incorporating small daily practices such as mindful, plant-based eating, natural movement, restorative sleep, stress management, deep social relationships, time for spiritual reflection, connection to nature, simple living, and an attitude of gratitude and optimism can make a huge difference in your health, well-being, and longevity.

It's not just about living longer, but about living with more quality, purpose, joy, and balance. The world's long-lived people haven't followed magic formulas; they've cultivated lifestyles that prioritize authenticity and vitality.

You too can start today. A small change, sustained with intention, can be the beginning of a lasting transformation.

Because in the end, the real secret to a long and full life isn't doing more, but living better.

Reflections on aging and living with purpose

Aging is an inevitable stage of life, but far from being a process that only brings limitations, it can be seen as an opportunity for reflection, personal growth, and the search for a deeper purpose.

Societies that value aging as a source of wisdom and experience teach us that the years should not be perceived as a burden, but as an accumulation of personal wealth and opportunities to continue learning and contributing.

Living with purpose as we age is key to maintaining a full and satisfying life. Having a clear sense of purpose—whether through work, family, volunteering, or personal development—gives direction to our actions and motivates us to stay active and engaged in life. This purpose not only drives us to take care of our physical health but also to nourish our minds and spirits.

Purpose in life can change over time, especially as we age. What once motivated us in our youth can transform as our priorities and perspectives evolve. However, the ability to adapt and find new sources of meaning is what makes the aging process a rich and meaningful time.

Staying active in your community, exploring new passions, or deepening your personal relationships are effective ways to continue finding meaning, regardless of age.

In Blue Zones, where longevity is the norm, a sense of purpose is deeply rooted in everyday life. Long-lived people don't view old age as a time of inactivity, but rather as an opportunity to continue contributing to the well-being of others and themselves. This approach not only improves mental and emotional health but also has a positive impact on physical longevity.

Purposeful aging also invites us to reconsider the value of each stage of life. It reminds us that, despite the physical changes that may occur, what remains constant is our capacity to learn, grow, and connect with others.

Finding purpose in aging leads us to live each day with intention, gratitude, and optimism, accepting the aging process as a natural and valuable part of the human experience.

In short, aging and purposeful living are intertwined, offering the opportunity to continue building a full and meaningful life, regardless of age. Living purposefully gives us a reason to stay active, nurture our relationships, and maintain a positive approach to challenges, which can ultimately contribute to greater longevity and well-being.

Recommended Reading

Below are some recommended readings that address topics related to longevity, health, and a Blue Zones lifestyle:

1. "The Blue Zones: 9 Lessons for Living Longer From the People Who've Lived the Longest" – Dan Buettner

This is the key book that introduced the world to the concept of Blue Zones. Dan Buettner, an explorer and writer for National Geographic, studied the regions of the world where people live the longest and with the best quality of life. It offers practical, science-based lessons for applying Blue Zone habits to modern life.

2. "Ikigai: The Japanese Secret to a Long and Happy Life" – Héctor García and Francesc Miralles

This book delves into the Japanese concept of ikigai, or "purpose," one of the fundamental principles of longevity in Okinawa, Japan. The authors explore how discovering your purpose in life can help you live a longer, more meaningful, and happier life.

3. "How Not to Die: Discover the Foods Scientifically Proven to Prevent and Reverse Disease" – Michael Greger, MD

This book focuses on the connection between nutrition and chronic disease prevention. Dr. Greger explains how a plant-based diet can not only improve health but also prolong life. It's an excellent read to understand the impact of natural and local foods on longevity.

4. "The Longevity Diet: Discover the New Science Behind Stem Cell Activation and Regeneration to Slow Aging, Fight Disease, and Optimize Weight" – Dr. Valter Longo

Dr. Valter Longo investigates the benefits of calorie restriction and intermittent fasting, common practices in some Blue Zones. This book offers science-based strategies to promote a longer, healthier life through diet and lifestyle.

5. "The Art of Simple Living: 100 Daily Practices from a Japanese Zen Monk for a Lifetime of Calm and Joy" – Shunmyo Masuno

This book explores simplicity and calm as keys to a more fulfilling and long life. Inspired by the principles of Zen philosophy, it teaches how small daily practices can reduce stress and promote mental and emotional well-being—essential elements of the Blue Zones.

6. "Outliers: The Story of Success" – Malcolm Gladwell

While not exclusively focused on longevity, Malcolm Gladwell's Outliers examines the key factors that influence success and excellence in life, including community and environment, which are principles that also underpin the Blue Zones. This read offers insight into how certain environments and lifestyles influence well-being and longevity.

7. "The Blue Zones Kitchen: 100 Recipes to Live to 100" – Dan Buettner

This book is a practical continuation of the study of the Blue Zones, focusing on traditional recipes from these regions. In addition to nutritional secrets, it offers concrete ideas for incorporating a plant-based diet, Blue Zone style, into your daily life.

8. "The Happiness Advantage: How a Positive Brain Fuels Success in Work and Life" – Shawn Achor

This book addresses how emotional and mental well-being, often promoted in Blue Zones through social connection and stress management, has a positive impact on longevity. Shawn Achor presents techniques for maintaining a positive attitude, which has been shown to prolong life and improve its quality.

9. "Why We Sleep: Unlocking the Power of Sleep and Dreams" – Matthew Walker

Sleep quality is another key factor in longevity. Matthew Walker explains the importance of rest and how restorative sleep can prevent disease and improve overall health. This book complements the Blue Zones approach to the importance of regular rest and relaxation.

10. "Atomic Habits: An Easy & Proven Way to Build Good Habits & Break Bad Ones" – James Clear

This book provides a practical approach to forming healthy habits that contribute to long-term well-being. Applying the Blue Zone principles in your daily life requires creating small, sustainable habits, and this book will teach you how to do this effectively.

These recommended reads are an excellent way to delve deeper into the secrets of longevity and learn how Blue Zone habits can be applied to improve health and well-being in everyday life. From mindful eating to stress management and discovering your life purpose, each book offers a unique perspective on how to live longer and better.

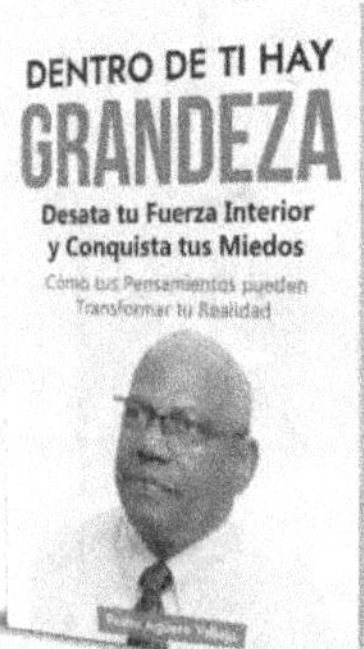

DENTRO DE TI HAY
GRANDEZA
Desata tu Fuerza Interior
y Conquista tus Miedos
Cómo tus Pensamientos pueden
Transformar tu Realidad
Pedro Agüero Vallejo

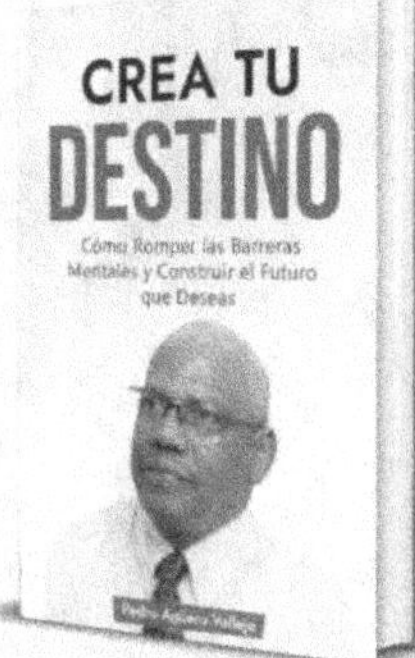

CREA TU
DESTINO
Cómo Romper las Barreras
Mentales y Construir el Futuro
que Deseas
Pedro Agüero Vallejo

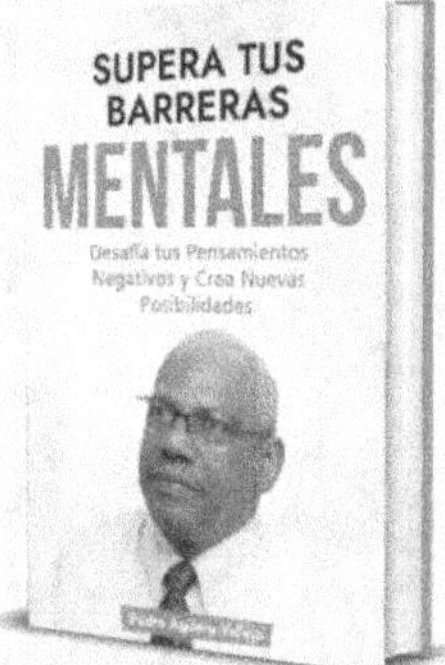

SUPERA TUS
BARRERAS
MENTALES
Desafía tus Pensamientos
Negativos y Crea Nuevas
Posibilidades
Pedro Agüero Vallejo

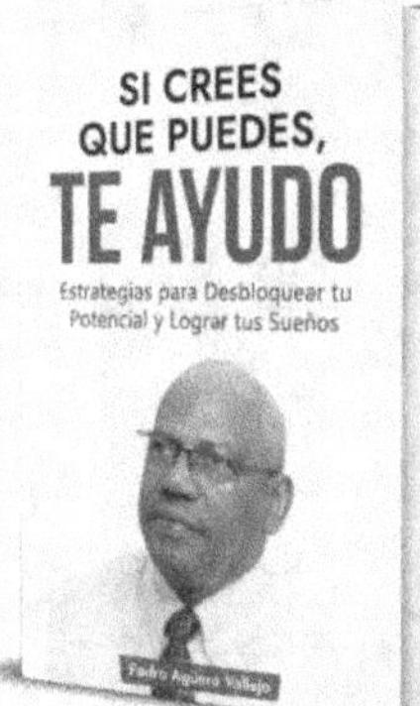

SI CREES
QUE PUEDES,
TE AYUDO
Estrategias para Desbloquear tu
Potencial y Lograr tus Sueños
Pedro Agüero Vallejo

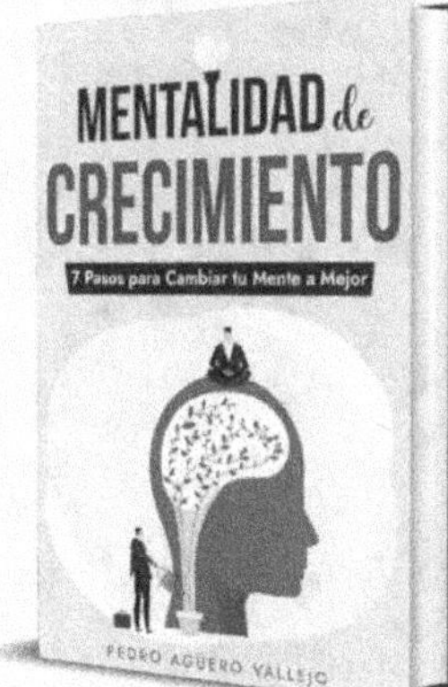

MENTALIDAD de
CRECIMIENTO
7 Pasos para Cambiar tu Mente a Mejor
PEDRO AGÜERO VALLEJO

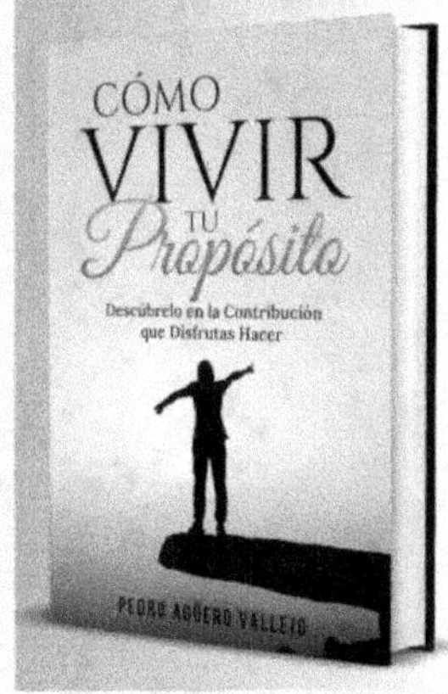

CÓMO
VIVIR
TU
Propósito
Descúbrelo en la Contribución
que Disfrutas Hacer
PEDRO AGÜERO VALLEJO

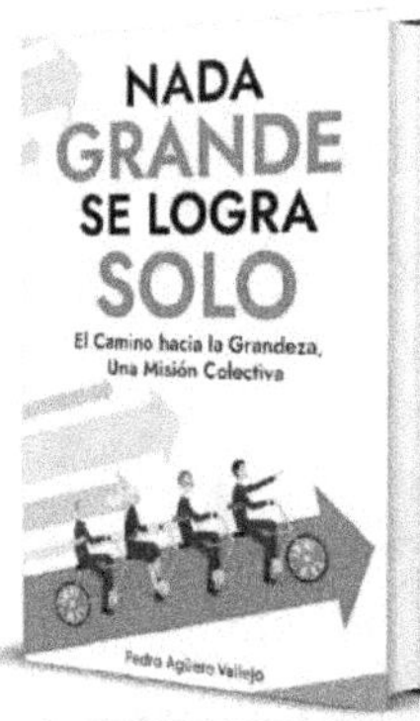

NADA
GRANDE
SE LOGRA
SOLO
El Camino hacia la Grandeza,
Una Misión Colectiva
Pedro Agüero Vallejo

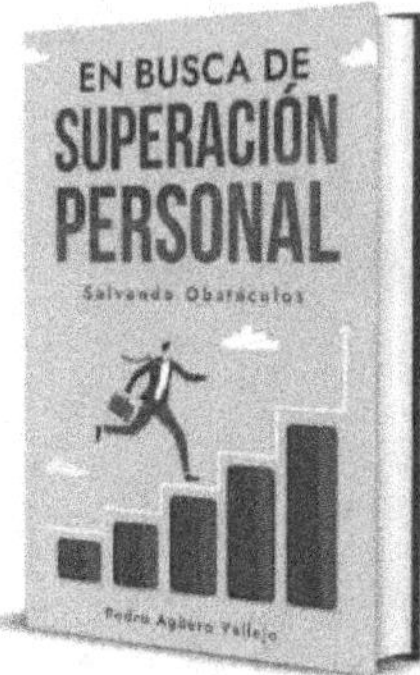

EN BUSCA DE
SUPERACIÓN
PERSONAL
Salvando Obstáculos
Pedro Agüero Vallejo

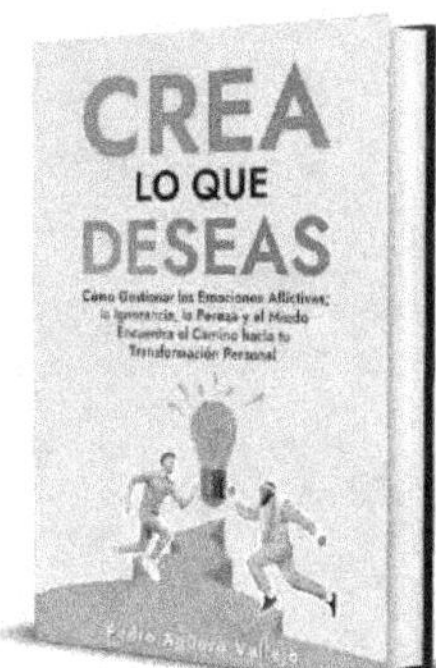

CREA
LO QUE
DESEAS
Cómo Gestionar las Emociones Aflictivas:
la Ignorancia, la Pereza y el Miedo
Encuentra el Camino hacia tu
Transformación Personal
Pedro Agüero Vallejo

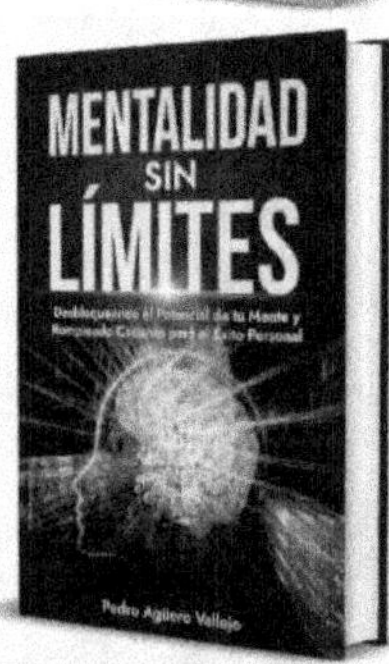

MENTALIDAD
SIN
LÍMITES
Desbloquea el Potencial de tu Mente y
Rompiendo Creencias para el Éxito Personal
Pedro Agüero Vallejo

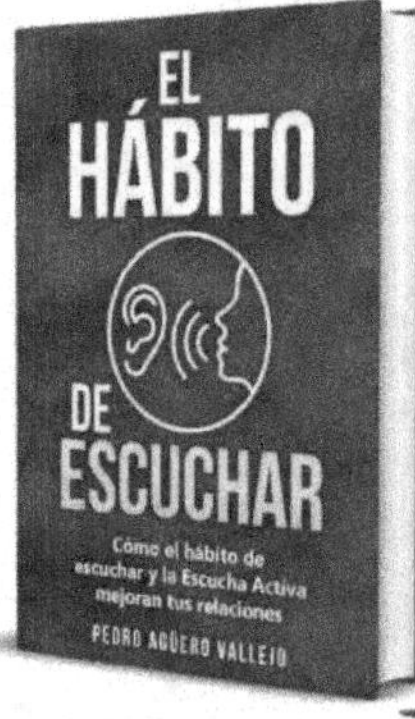

EL
HÁBITO
DE
ESCUCHAR
Cómo el hábito de
escuchar y la Escucha Activa
mejoran tus relaciones
PEDRO AGÜERO VALLEJO

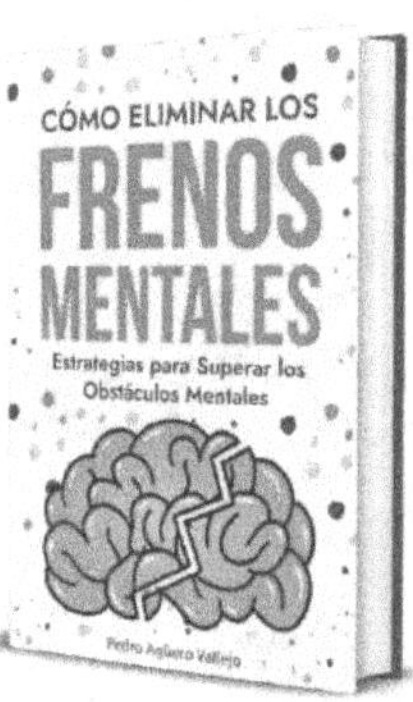

CÓMO ELIMINAR LOS
FRENOS
MENTALES
Estrategias para Superar los
Obstáculos Mentales
Pedro Agüero Vallejo

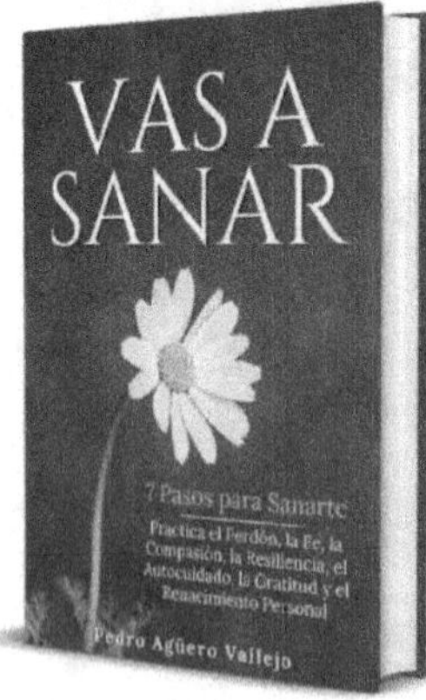

VAS A
SANAR
7 Pasos para Sanarte
Practica el Perdón, la Fe, la
Compasión, la Resiliencia, el
Autocuidado, la Gratitud y el
Renacimiento Personal
Pedro Agüero Vallejo

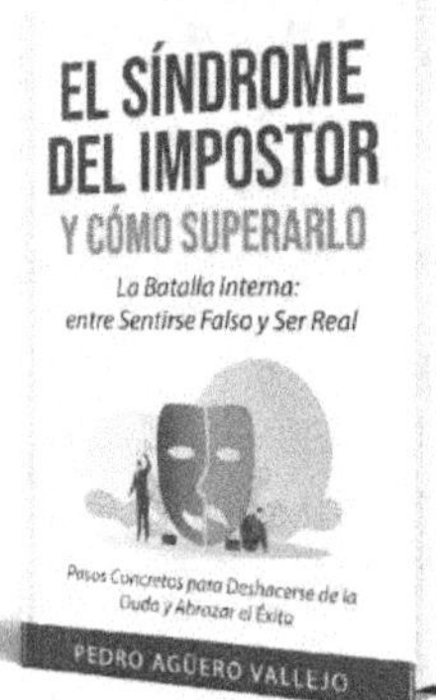

EL SÍNDROME
DEL IMPOSTOR
Y CÓMO SUPERARLO
La Batalla Interna:
entre Sentirse Falso y Ser Real
Pasos Concretos para Deshacerse de la
Duda y Abrazar el Éxito
PEDRO AGÜERO VALLEJO

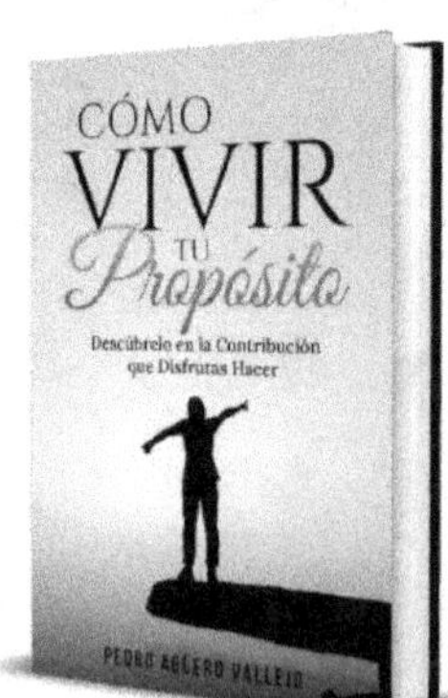

CÓMO
VIVIR
TU
Propósito
Descúbrelo en la Contribución
que Disfrutas Hacer
PEDRO AGÜERO VALLEJO

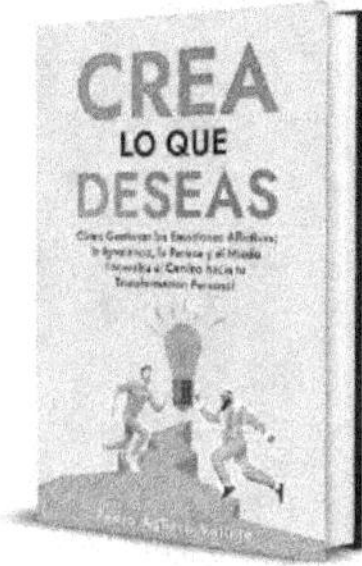

CREA
LO QUE
DESEAS
Pedro Agüero Vallejo

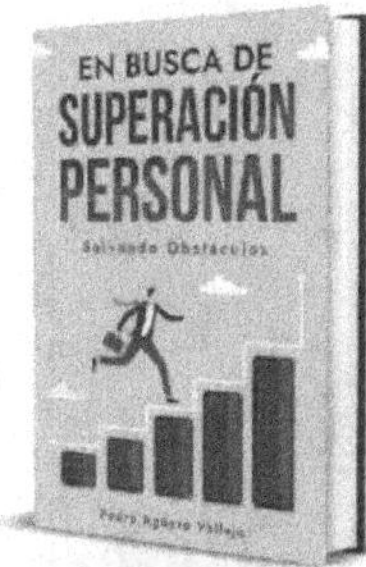

EN BUSCA DE
SUPERACIÓN
PERSONAL
Salvando Obstáculos
Pedro Agüero Vallejo

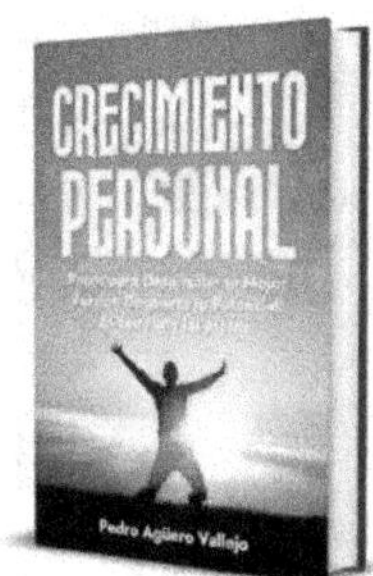

CRECIMIENTO
PERSONAL
Pedro Agüero Vallejo

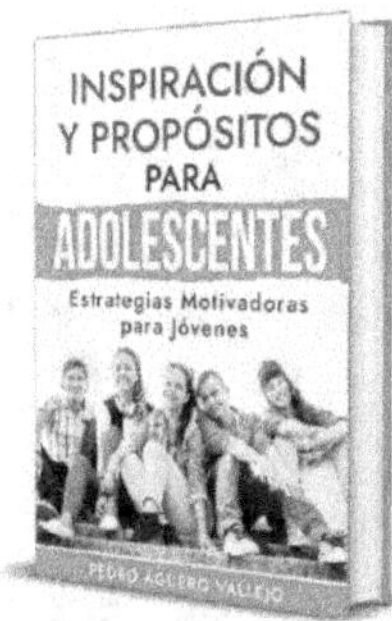

INSPIRACIÓN
Y PROPÓSITOS
PARA
ADOLESCENTES
Estrategias Motivadoras
para Jóvenes
PEDRO AGÜERO VALLEJO

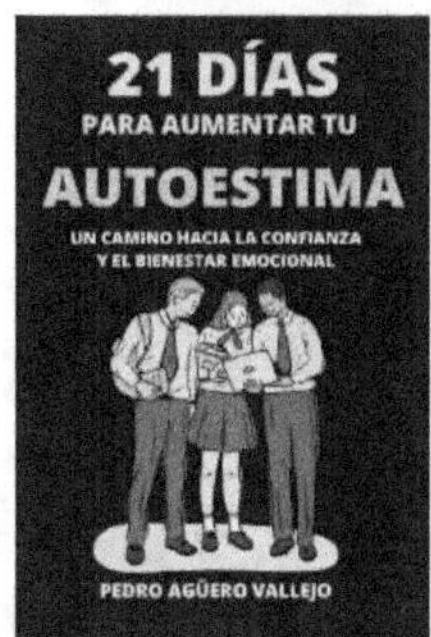

21 DÍAS
PARA AUMENTAR TU
AUTOESTIMA
UN CAMINO HACIA LA CONFIANZA
Y EL BIENESTAR EMOCIONAL
PEDRO AGÜERO VALLEJO

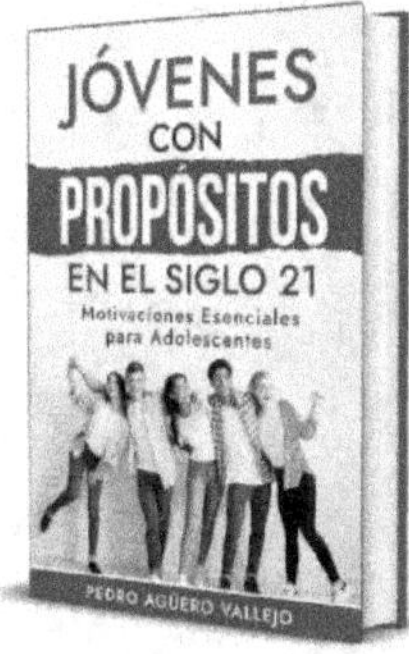

JÓVENES
CON
PROPÓSITOS
EN EL SIGLO 21
Motivaciones Esenciales
para Adolescentes
PEDRO AGÜERO VALLEJO

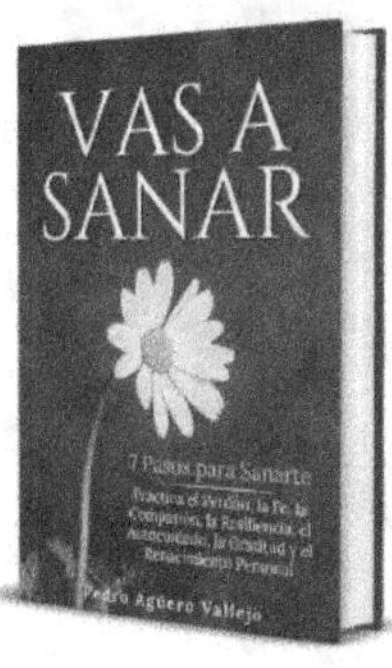

VAS A
SANAR
7 Pasos para Sanarte
Pedro Agüero Vallejo

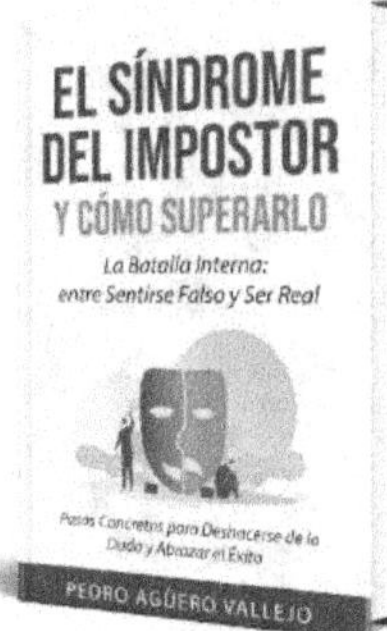

EL SÍNDROME
DEL IMPOSTOR
Y CÓMO SUPERARLO
La Batalla Interna:
entre Sentirse Falso y Ser Real
Pasos Concretos para Deshacerse de la
Duda y Abrazar el Éxito
PEDRO AGÜERO VALLEJO

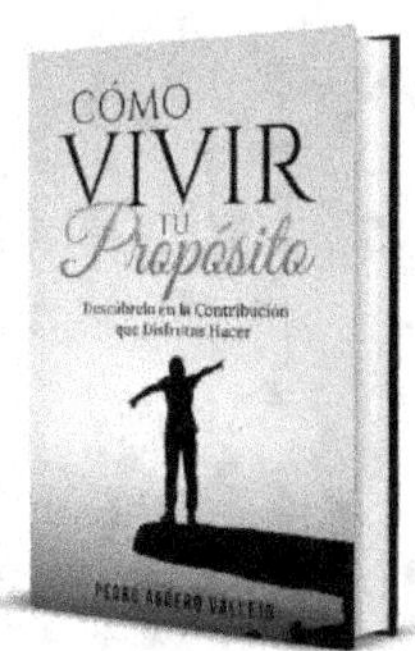

CÓMO
VIVIR
TU
Propósito
Descúbrelo en la Contribución
que Disfrutas Hacer
PEDRO AGÜERO VALLEJO

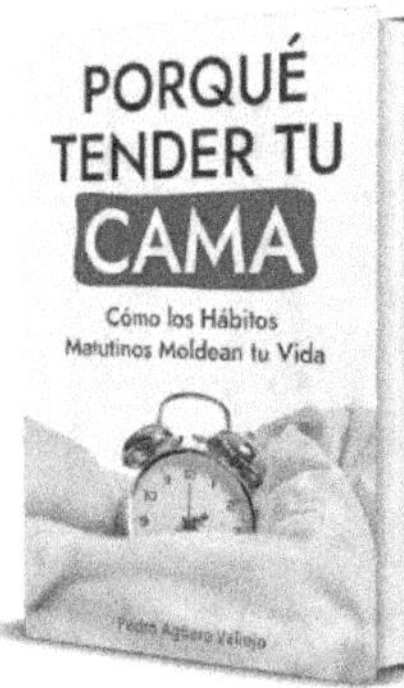
PORQUÉ
TENDER TU
CAMA
Cómo los Hábitos
Matutinos Moldean tu Vida
Pedro Agüero Vallejo

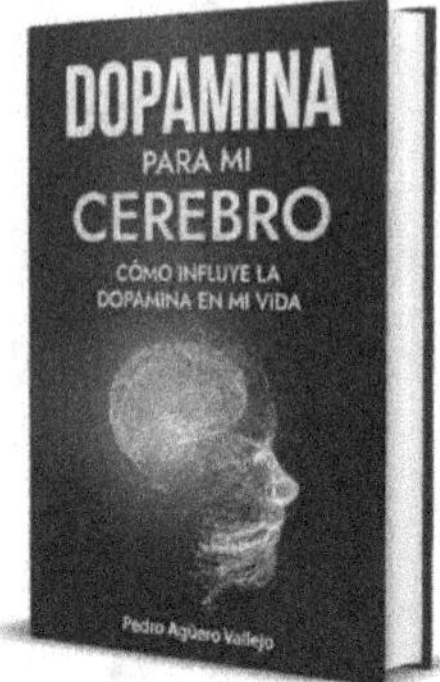
DOPAMINA
PARA MI
CEREBRO
CÓMO INFLUYE LA
DOPAMINA EN MI VIDA
Pedro Agüero Vallejo

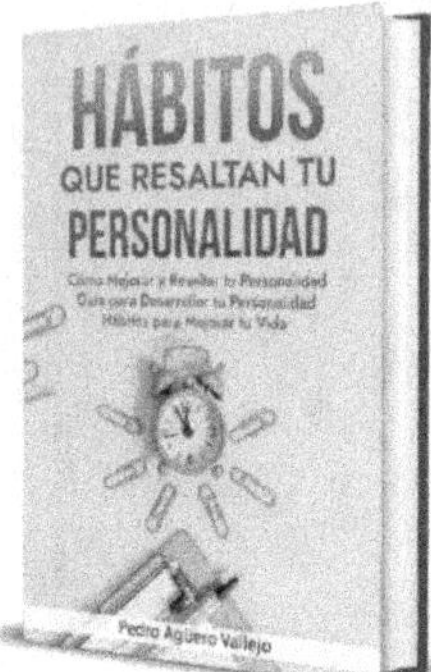
HÁBITOS
QUE RESALTAN TU
PERSONALIDAD
Cómo Mejorar y Resaltar tu Personalidad
Guía para Desarrollar tu Personalidad
Hábitos para Mejorar tu Vida
Pedro Agüero Vallejo

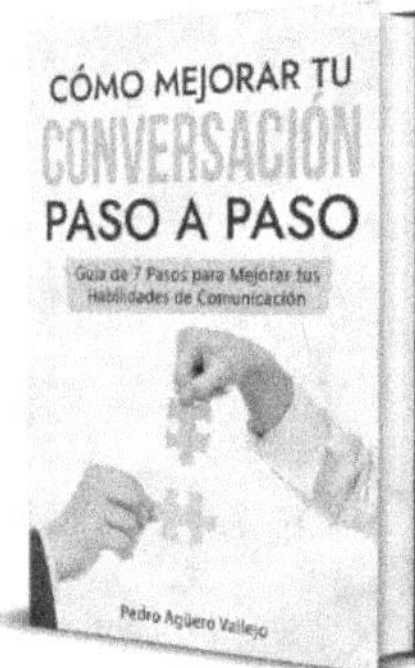
CÓMO MEJORAR TU
CONVERSACIÓN
PASO A PASO
Guía de 7 Pasos para Mejorar tus
Habilidades de Comunicación
Pedro Agüero Vallejo

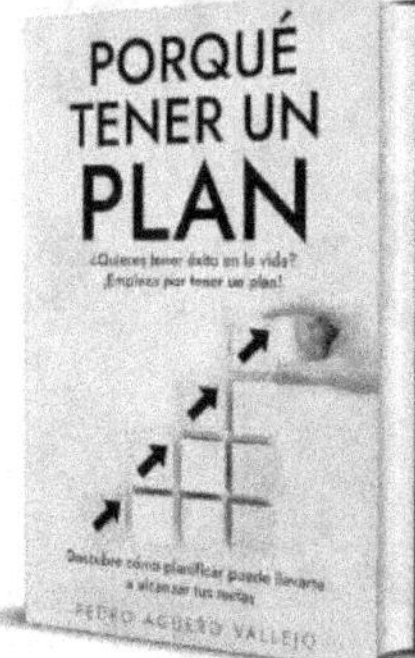
PORQUÉ
TENER UN
PLAN
¿Quieres tener éxito en la vida?
¡Empieza por tener un plan!
Descubre cómo planificar puede llevarte
a alcanzar tus metas
PEDRO AGÜERO VALLEJO

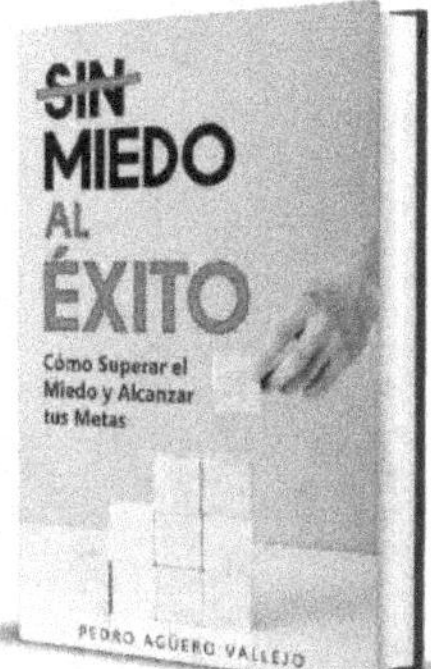
SIN
MIEDO
AL
ÉXITO
Cómo Superar el
Miedo y Alcanzar
tus Metas
PEDRO AGÜERO VALLEJO

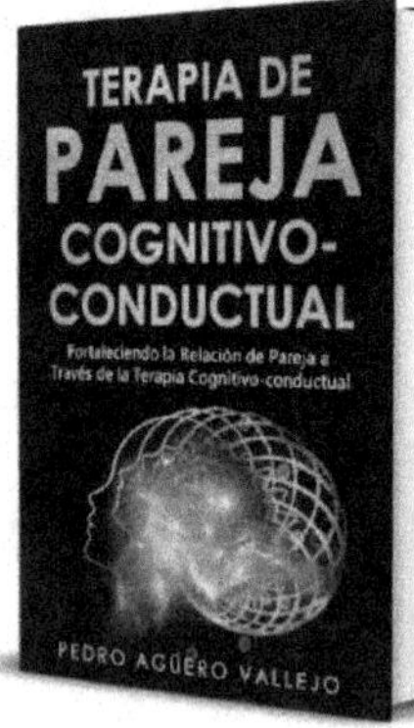
TERAPIA DE
PAREJA
COGNITIVO-
CONDUCTUAL
Fortaleciendo la Relación de Pareja a
Través de la Terapia Cognitivo-conductual
PEDRO AGÜERO VALLEJO

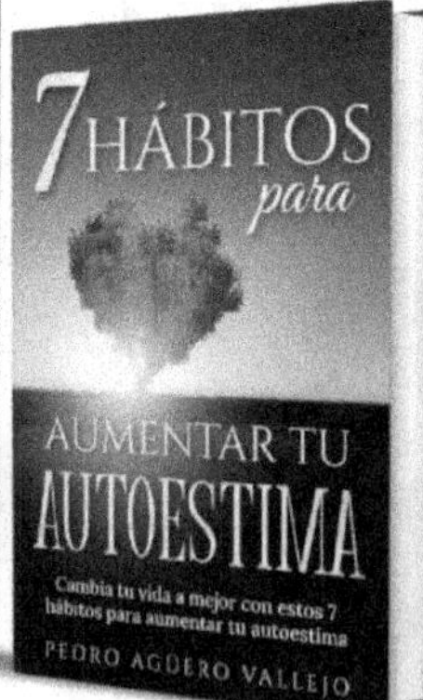
7 HÁBITOS
para
AUMENTAR TU
AUTOESTIMA
Cambia tu vida a mejor con estos 7
hábitos para aumentar tu autoestima
PEDRO AGÜERO VALLEJO

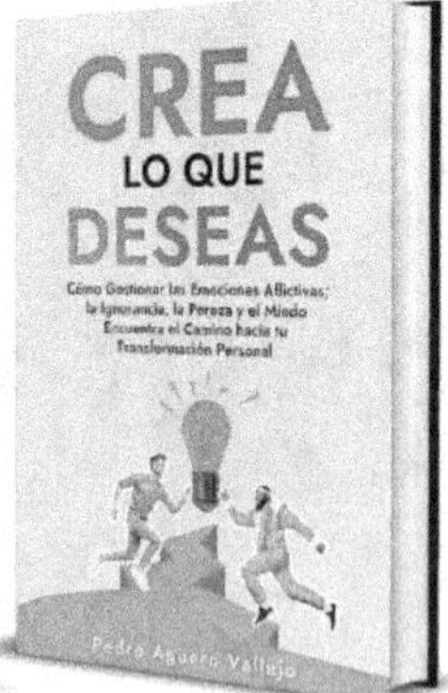
CREA
LO QUE
DESEAS
Cómo Gestionar las Emociones Aflictivas:
la Ignorancia, la Pereza y el Miedo
Encuentra el Camino hacia tu
Transformación Personal
Pedro Agüero Vallejo

Todos mis libros